Fiber-Reinforced Composites in Clinical Dentistry

FIBER-REINFORCED
COMPOSITES
IN CLINICAL DENTISTRY

Martin A. Freilich, DDS
Department of Prosthodontics and Operative Dentistry
University of Connecticut
School of Dental Medicine
Farmington, Connecticut

Jonathan C. Meiers, DMD, MS
Department of Prosthodontics and Operative Dentistry
University of Connecticut
School of Dental Medicine
Farmington, Connecticut

Jacqueline P. Duncan, DMD, MDSc
Department of Prosthodontics and Operative Dentistry
University of Connecticut
School of Dental Medicine
Farmington, Connecticut

A. Jon Goldberg, PhD
Department of Prosthodontics and Operative Dentistry
Center for Biomaterials
University of Connecticut
School of Dental Medicine
Farmington, Connecticut

Quintessence Publishing Co, Inc
Chicago, Berlin, London, Tokyo, Paris, Barcelona, São Paulo,
Moscow, Prague, and Warsaw

Library of Congress Cataloging-in-Publication Data

Fiber-reinforced composites in clinical dentistry / Martin A. Freilich … [et al.].
    p. ; cm.
    Includes bibliographical references and index.
    ISBN 0-86715-373-3
    1. Fibrous composites in dentistry. I. Freilich, Martin A.
    [DNLM: 1. Dental Materials. 2. Composite Resins. 3. Dental Prosthesis Design. WU
190 F443 1999]
    RK655.3 .F53 1999
    617.6'95—dc21   99-046512

© 2000 Quintessence Publishing Co, Inc

Quintessence Publishing Co, Inc
551 Kimberly Drive
Carol Stream, Illinois 60188

Editor: Lisa C. Bywaters
Design/Production: Michael Shanahan

Printed in Hong Kong

Contents

The authors dedicate this book to their families, for their love and support, and to their mentors, who have helped them achieve success in their professional careers.

Preface

■ Several years ago our research group at the University of Connecticut became intrigued by the question of why fiber-reinforced composite materials, which had been used successfully in a variety of commercial applications, were not more widely used in dentistry. After a careful review of the literature and some preliminary research, it became clear to us that the use of fiber-reinforced composites in existing dental applications was compromised by three important limitations: low fiber content, insufficient fiber wetting, and the difficulty of manipulating free fibers. Through the development of pre-impregnation technology, which has served as the primary focus of our research group over the past 10 years, these problems have been largely overcome.

Fiber-reinforced materials have highly favorable mechanical properties, and their strength-to-weight ratios are superior to those of most alloys. When compared to metals they offer many other advantages as well, including noncorrosiveness, translucency, good bonding properties, and ease of repair. Since they also offer the potential for chairside and laboratory fabrication, it is not surprising that fiber-reinforced composites have potential for use in many applications in dentistry.

While early clinical trials validated many of our concepts, the need for improved laboratory and clinical procedures soon became apparent. Some procedures were refined, and additional applications were studied in both the laboratory and the clinic. Our research group has collaborated with the Jeneric/Pentron company to develop a pre-impregnated, fiber-reinforced composite substructure material tradenamed FibreKor. Ivoclar has used a similar pre-impregnation technology to produce a fiber-reinforced composite material, also for use in fixed prosthodontics, tradenamed Vectris. Both of these commercially available systems are being used by a growing number of dental practitioners.

To realize the full potential of using fiber-reinforced composites, it is essential that the clinician and laboratory technician understand concepts of tooth preparation and framework design. In this book we have attempted to present the clinical information necessary to allow the reader to identify appropriate cases, select well-suited materials, and carry out related procedures. The publisher has graciously encouraged the liberal use of clinical photographs and diagrams to make these details clear. At the same time, we have provided background information and other details about the materials themselves so that the practitioner may appreciate the rationale for their use in various clinical situations. Every effort has been made to include the most widely used products from different manufacturers along with the different characteristics and relative advantages of each.

The field of fiber-reinforced composites continues to expand at a rapid pace. New products are being introduced even at this writing. We hope that the procedures described in this book will allow clinicians to incorporate the use of these materials into everyday practice and that the background will provide a basis for understanding future products and procedures.

The authors would like to acknowledge the early scientific contributions made by Dr Charles J. Burstone to the development of fiber-reinforced composites, including his ideas for potential clinical applications in dentistry. Dr James V. Altieri's work with an early FRC is also acknowledged. Dr Ajit Karmaker was an important member of the group that developed the first light-polymerized formulation, and continues to be of assistance to the authors.

They also gratefully acknowledge Connecticut Innovations, Inc, whose financial support of university-industry collaborations enabled important development and commercialization efforts. Several companies producing fiber-reinforced composites for dentistry—Ribbond, Glasspan, and Kerr—provided materials, freely discussed their technologies, and offered useful comments about this and earlier publications. Additionally, Ivoclar, Inc graciously provided materials, equipment, and participation in the Targis/Vectris Training Program.

A special acknowledgment goes to the Jeneric/Pentron Corporation for the comprehensive collaborative relationship they have maintained with the University of Connecticut Health Center to help bring fiber reinforcement to the dental profession.

The authors also express their gratitude to Dr Howard E. Strassler for contributing clinical photographs and text for chapter 4; Dr Thomas N. Trinkner, Dr Bruce Marcucci, and Dr Anil Patel for contributing clinical photographs; Mr Everett Pearson and TPI Composites for contributing photographs of their fiber-reinforced products; and Dr Reza Kazemi for contributing illustrations.

Finally, the authors would like to thank Ms Diane Kosis, MPH Coordinator of the University of Connecticut Clinical Dental Research Center, and Ms Shirley Carrolla and Ms Kimberly Haser, laboratory staff of the University of Connecticut Biomaterials Center.

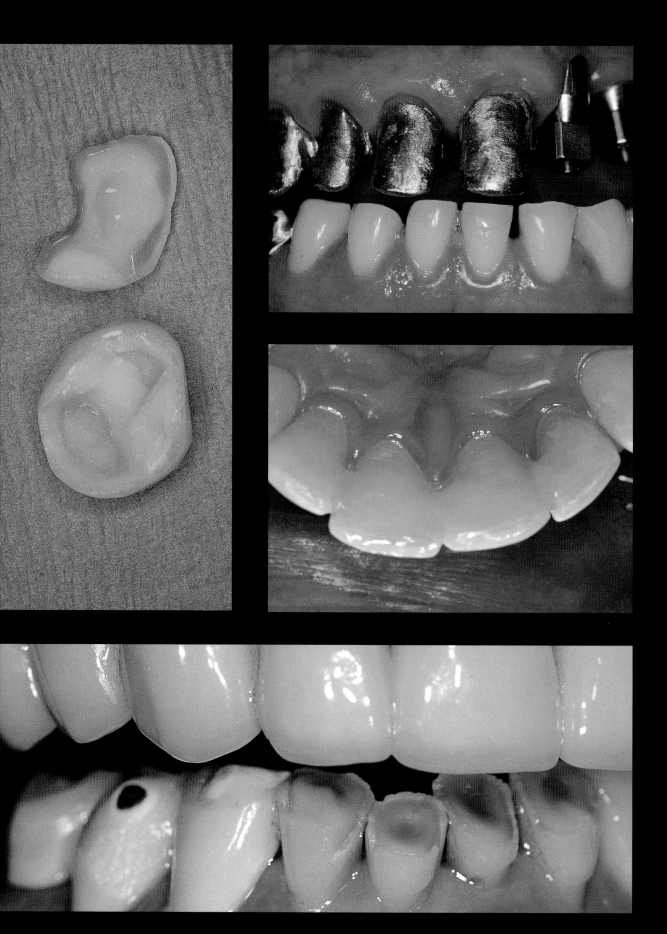

Rationale for the Clinical Use of Fiber-reinforced Composites

■ The technology and materials available to today's restorative dentists offer various solutions to many complex problems. Missing tooth structure can be replaced through the use of adhesives or metal-ceramic crowns (Fig 1-1), and missing teeth can be replaced with any of a variety of fixed prostheses supported by teeth (Fig 1-2) or implants (Fig 1-3). Porcelain-fused-to-metal substructures continue to be a mainstay of fixed prosthodontics, and polymethyl methacrylate (PMMA) polymer remains the material of choice for complete denture bases.

As popular and successful as these materials are, they exhibit shortcomings that frequently cause clinical problems:

1. The metal alloys used to make substructures that reinforce crowns and fixed prostheses are strong and rigid, but they are not esthetic (Figs 1-4 and 1-5). Furthermore, the base metal alloys commonly used in clinical practice may corrode and some patients have an allergic reaction to them.[2] Certain components of some base metal alloys may even pose acute and chronic health hazards to laboratory personnel.[8,9]

2. Ceramic materials such as porcelain may exhibit good optical qualities, but they are also brittle and hard, they have the potential to lose structural integrity (Fig 1-6), and they sometimes abrade or fracture the opposing teeth (Fig 1-7).

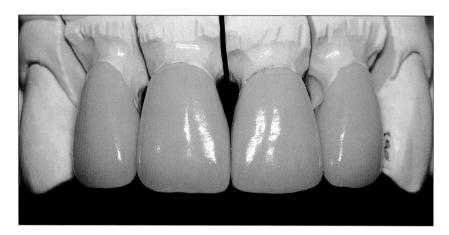

Fig 1-1 Metal-ceramic crowns seated on a working cast prior to delivery.

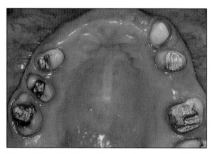

Fig 1-2a Multi-unit metal-ceramic fixed partial denture illustrating final tooth preparations.

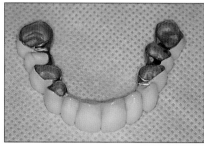

Fig 1-2b Underside view of the prosthesis.

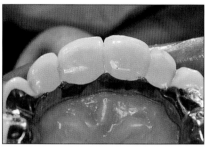

Fig 1-2c Prosthesis after placement in the mouth.

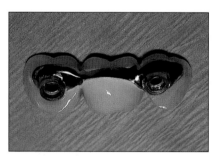

Fig 1-3 Three-unit posterior metal-ceramic implant prosthesis, prior to placement.

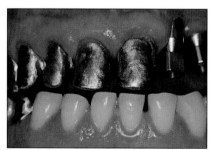

Fig 1-4 Metal alloy copings used as substructure for metal-ceramic crowns, at try-in appointment.

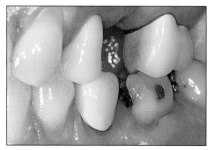

Fig 1-5a Maxillary and mandibular posterior metal-ceramic crowns exhibiting cervical metal collars.

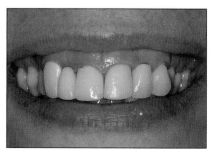

Fig 1-5b Maxillary anterior FPD exhibiting cervical metal collars.

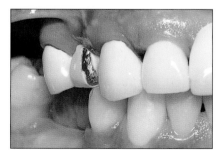

Fig 1-6 Metal-ceramic FPD with a fractured porcelain veneer.

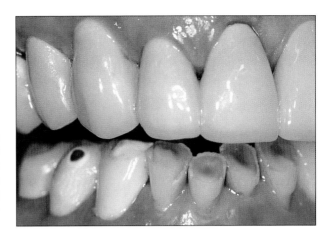

Fig 1-7 Sequelae resulting from use of hard, brittle porcelain veneer. Severely abraded mandibular anterior teeth oppose the porcelain and porcelain-metal junction of metal-ceramic crowns. Mandibular metal-ceramic crowns have a partially abraded porcelain veneer and a higher-than-desired value (too bright) because of inadequate thickness of body porcelain covering opaque porcelain.

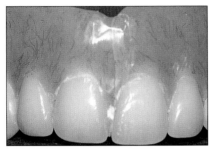 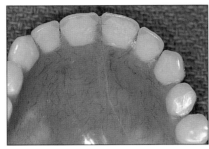 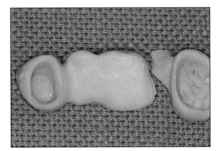

Figs 1-8a and 1-8b Failure of PMMA polymer, with fractured maxillary complete denture.   **Fig 1-8c** Broken provisional FPD.

3. The opaque porcelains used to mask the metal substructure are themselves not esthetic, and they require a minimum thickness of coverage to obtain an acceptable result (see Fig 1-7).

4. The acrylic polymer materials such as methyl methacrylate that are used to make removable and provisional fixed prostheses offer desirable handling qualities and physical properties, but they are susceptible to fracture in many clinical circumstances (Fig 1-8).

Some clinical conditions have never been managed satisfactorily with available materials or techniques:

1. Attempts to stabilize unrestored or minimally restored mobile teeth with the use of amalgams or restorative composites, whether with or without metal wire, frequently prove unsatisfactory. The use of cast metal plates to stabilize these teeth has been expensive, technique-sensitive, and unesthetic (Fig 1-9). The use of metal-ceramic full-coverage crowns as a splint requires removal of substantial healthy tooth structure and a large financial investment in return for teeth with a somewhat questionable prognosis.

2. The search for an immediate chairside tooth replacement continues. In the past, conservative replacement techniques have used pontics from extracted teeth,[1,5,11] acrylic teeth,[3,10,12] and resin composite.[6,11,13,14] These pontics, which are attached to adjacent abutment teeth using an acid-etch, resin-bonding technique and composite with or without wire, generally have a short life.

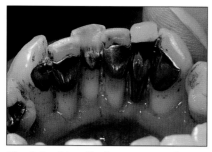

Fig 1-9a Mandibular cast metal peri-odontal splints.

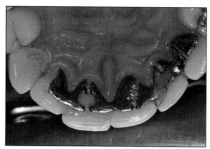

Fig 1-9b Maxillary cast metal periodontal splints.

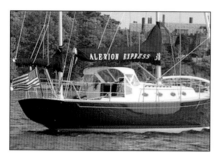

Fig 1-10 High-quality sailboat with glass fiber–reinforced hull. (Courtesy of TPI Composites Inc.)

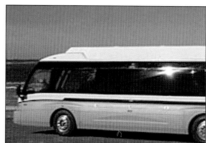

Fig 1-11 Bus with glass fiber–reinforced body. (Courtesy of TPI Composites Inc.)

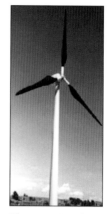

Fig 1-12 Modern windmill with carbon fiber–reinforced blades. (Courtesy of TPI Composites Inc.)

Applications for Fiber-reinforced Composites Outside Dentistry

Fiber-reinforced composites (FRCs) have the potential to remedy many of the structural and esthetic problems described above. The use of these materials is new to dentistry, but their many desirable characteristics have found application in a number of industries outside dentistry. Recreational boat hulls (Fig 1-10) as well as many other components used in the boating industry, such as masts and rudders, are now routinely made with FRCs. High-quality buses (Fig 1-11) and large modern windmills (Fig 1-12) are also made with fiber-reinforced materials.

Fiber-reinforced materials have good overall mechanical properties, and their strength-to-weight ratios are superior to those of most alloys. Noncorrosive properties, potential translucency, radiolucency, good bonding properties, and ease of repair are additional features that make these materials advantageous compared to metals. Given that they also offer the potential for chairside and laboratory fabrication, it is not surprising that FRCs have many applications in dentistry.

Using Fiber-reinforced Composites in Dentistry

Dentists work with composites all the time. Restorative composites consist of particles of quartz or glass held together by a resinous matrix. Dentists use these "particulate" composites to restore defects in a single tooth or as a veneer material for a tooth or prosthesis. Fiber-reinforced composites consist of fiber material held together by a resinous matrix. As noted above, they offer good flexure strength and other physical qualities required in a prosthesis substructure material.[4,7]

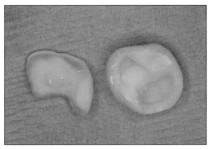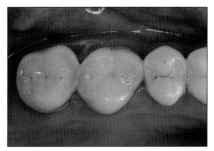

Figs 1-13a and 1-13b Maxillary left first and second molars restored with FRC crowns made of Targis/Vectris (Ivoclar North America). (Courtesy of Dr Thomas Trinkner.)

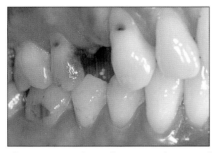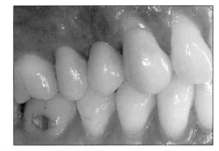

Figs 1-14a and 1-14b Intraoral views of full-coverage FRC FPD from maxillary right second premolar to canine made of Scupture/FibreKor (Jeneric/Pentron). (a) Pretreatment. (b) Posttreatment.

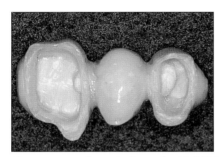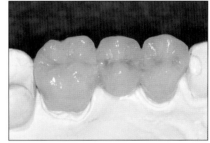

Figs 1-15a and 1-15b Posterior FRC FPD. (a) Underside view. (b) Occlusal aspect.

Some FRC substructure materials retain a sticky, oxygen-inhibited surface layer that allows for direct chemical bonding with a veneer composite, thereby eliminating the need for mechanical retention associated with a metal substructure. Fiber-reinforced composite materials can be used to make frameworks for crowns (Fig 1-13), anterior or posterior fixed prostheses (Figs 1-14 and 1-15), chairside tooth replacements (Fig 1-16), and appliances such as periodontal splints (Fig 1-17).

For a single crown or fixed partial denture (FPD), the FRC framework replaces the classic metal framework of a porcelain-fused-to-metal prosthesis, while the application of a particulate composite over this FRC framework corresponds to that of porcelain over a traditional metal substructure. The FRC framework provides strength and rigidity beneath the outer layer of particulate composite. This two-component polymer prosthesis, shown in Fig 1-18, combines the best characteristics of the FRC

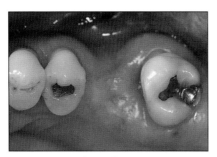
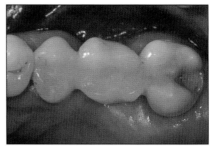

Figs 1-16a and 1-16b Intraoral views of a chairside-fabricated FRC FPD from maxillary left second premolar to second molar. (a) Pretreatment. (b) Posttreatment.

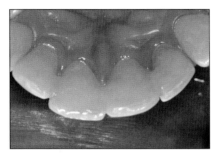
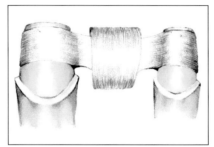
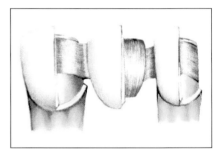

Fig 1-17 Chairside-fabricated FRC periodontal splint made on the lingual aspect of maxillary anterior teeth.

Fig 1-18 Illustration of the FRC substructure for an anterior 3-unit FPD. (Special thanks to Dr Reza Kazemi.)

Fig 1-19 Illustration of the FRC substructure partially overlayed with covering particulate composite, showing the support that the substructure provides for the composite veneer. (Special thanks to Dr Reza Kazemi.)

(strength and rigidity) with the best characteristics of the particulate composite (wear resistance and esthetics). Since it can be bonded directly to abutment teeth, such a prosthesis is useful where there is less-than-optimal retention and resistance form.

Essential Clinical Skills

Fiber-reinforced materials have wide potential for application in a variety of clinical situations, but the clinician must understand the basic structure of these materials and the different types available. Awareness of the advantages and limitations of each type of FRC enables the clinician to select the best FRC material for each particular clinical circumstance.

For splints, crowns, and fixed prostheses, the clinician must be able to make FRC tooth preparations that allow the dental laboratory to place an adequate volume of FRC to make a durable, biocompatible framework and prosthesis. The clinician needs to understand framework design concepts because there is strong evidence that this is a crucial factor in the success or failure of a fiber-reinforced prosthesis. Lastly, the clinician must be able to perform techniques for luting an indirect prosthesis or fabricating a direct prosthesis or appliance. The chapters that follow are intended to provide these essential skills to the clinician and demonstrate many additional applications for this technology.

References

1. Antonson DE. Immediate temporary bridge using an extracted tooth. Dent Surv 1980;56:22–25.

2. Council on Dental Materials, Instruments, and Equipment. Report on base metal alloys for crown and bridge applications: Benefits and risks. J Am Dent Assoc 1985;111:479–483.

3. Davila JM, Gwinnett AV. Clinical and microscopic evaluation of a bridge using the acid-etch technique. J Dent Child 1978;45:228–232.

4. Freilich MA, Karmaker AC, Burstone CJ, Goldberg AJ. Flexure strength of fiber-reinforced composites designed for prosthodontic application [abstract 999]. J Dent Res 1997;76(special issue):138.

5. Ibsen RL. Fixed prosthetics with a natural crown pontic using an adhesive composite. J South Calif Dent Assoc 1973;41:100–102.

6. Jensen ME, Meiers JC. Resin-Bonded Retainers in Clinical Dentistry, vol 4. Philadelphia: Harper and Row, 1984:4–5.

7. Karmaker AC, DiBenedetto AT, Goldberg AJ. Fiber-reinforced composite materials for dental appliances. Presented at the Society of Plastic Engineers Annual Technical Conference, Indianapolis, 5–9 May 1996.

8. Moffa JP, Beck WD, Hoke AW. Allergic response to nickel-containing dental alloys [abstract 107]. J Dent Res 1977;56:1378.

9. Morris HF. Veterans Administration Cooperative Studies Project No. 147. IV. Biocompatibility of base metal alloys. J Dent 1987;56(special issue):B78.

10. Portnoy LL. Constructing a composite pontic in a single visit. Dent Surv 1973;49:20–23.

11. Simonsen RJ. Clinical Applications of the Acid Etch Technique. Chicago: Quintessence, 1978:71.

12. Simonsen RJ. The acid etch technique in fixed prostheses. An update. Quintessence Int 1980;9:33.

13. Simonsen R, Thompson V, Barrack G. Etched Cast Restorations: Clinical and Laboratory Techniques. Chicago: Quintessence, 1983.

14. Stolpa JB. An adhesive technique for small anterior fixed partial dentures. J Prosthet Dent 1975;34:513–519.

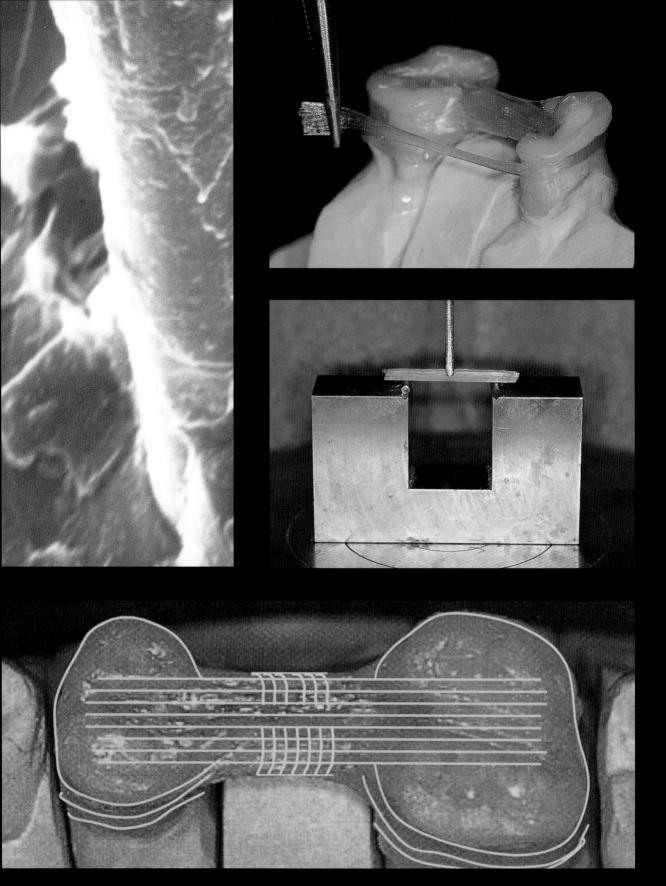

Composition, Architecture, and Mechanical Properties of Fiber-reinforced Composites

■ Fiber-reinforced composites (FRCs) are structural materials that have at least two distinct constituents. The reinforcing component provides strength and stiffness, while the surrounding matrix supports the reinforcement and provides workability. One of the constituents may be metal, ceramic, or polymer; in dental applications, polymeric or resin matrices reinforced with glass, polyethylene, or carbon fiber are most common. The fibers may be arranged in various configurations: "unidirectional" fibers (Fig 2-1)—long, continuous, and parallel—are the most popular, followed by braided and woven fibers (Fig 2-2). Typically, fibers are 7 to 10 μm in diameter and span the length of the prosthesis or appliance. By comparison, the particles used in standard restorative dental composites are 1 to 5 μm in diameter, or submicron in size (Fig 2-3).

The type of fiber used to make an FRC depends on how it is intended to be used and the characteristics that are needed for that purpose. Glass fibers of various kinds are commonly used in dental laboratory products, while polymeric reinforcements, such as polyethylene, are often used for chairside applications. Posts are made of carbon or glass fibers. Table 2-1 lists different types of fiber and the important mechanical and physical characteristics of each. The types of fiber and architecture found in various products are shown in Table 2-2; products are classified according to their clinical uses and whether the fiber bundles

Fig 2-1 Unidirectional fiber-reinforced composite.

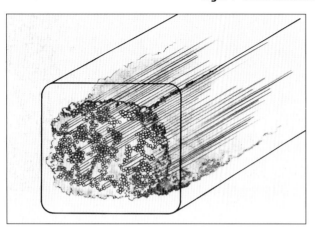

Fig 2-1a Schematic diagram.

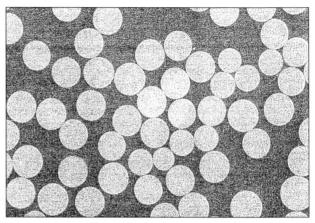

Fig 2-1b Scanning electron micrograph cross section of polished pontic region of FPD framework (FibreKor, Jeneric/Pentron).

Fig 2-2 Scanning electron micrographs of various fiber architectures.

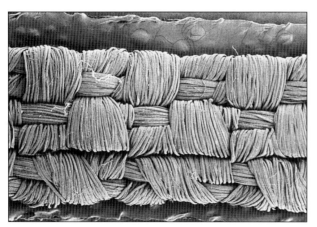

Fig 2-2a Woven polyethylene fibers (Ribbond, Ribbond).

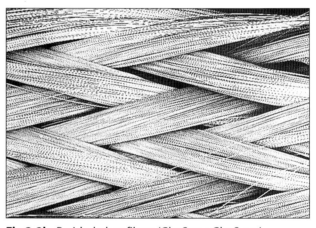

Fig 2-2b Braided glass fibers (GlasSpan, GlasSpan).

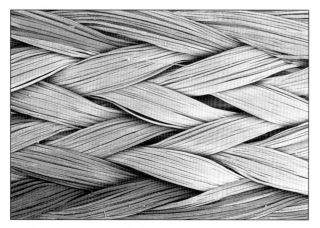

Fig 2-2c Braided polyethylene fibers (Connect, Kerr).

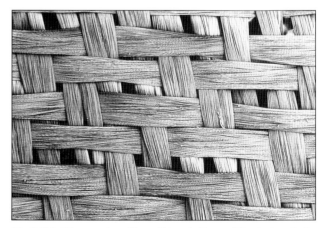

Fig 2-2d Woven glass fibers (Vectris Frame/Single, Ivoclar).

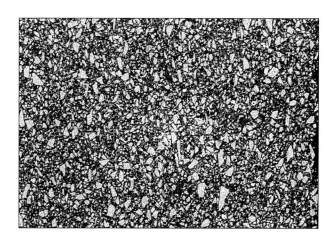

Fig 2-3 Scanning electron micrograph of restorative dental composite (Sculpture, Jeneric/Pentron).

Table 2-1 | Mechanical and physical properties of reinforcing fibers

	Tensile strength (MPa)	Tensile modulus of elasticity (GPa)	Elongation (%)	Density (g/cm^3)
E-glass	3,400	72	4.9	2.62
S-glass	4,500	85	5.7	2.50
Carbon/graphite	2,400–3,300	230–390	0.6–1.4	1.70–1.90
Aramid (Kevlar)	3,600–4,100	62–130	2.8–4.0	1.44
Polyethylene (Spectra 900)	2,600	117	3.5	0.97

Table 2-2 | Classification of fiber-reinforced composite dental products

Product	Company	Fiber type	Fiber architecture
Pre-impregnated, dental laboratory products			
FibreKor	Jeneric/Pentron	Glass	Unidirectional
Vectris pontic	Ivoclar	Glass	Unidirectional
Vectris frame and single	Ivoclar	Glass	Mesh
Pre-impregnated, chairside products			
Splint-It	Jeneric/Pentron	Glass	Unidirectional
Splint-It	Jeneric/Pentron	Glass	Weave
Splint-It	Jeneric/Pentron	Polyethylene	Weave
Impregnation required, chairside products			
Connect	Kerr	Polyethylene	Braid
DVA Fibers	Dental Ventures	Polyethylene	Unidirectional
Fiber-Splint	Inter Dental Distributors	Glass	Weave
Fibreflex	Biocomp	Kevlar	Unidirectional
GlasSpan	GlasSpan	Glass	Braid
Ribbond	Ribbond	Polyethylene	Leno Weave
Pre-impregnated prefabricated posts			
C-Post	Bisco	Carbon	Unidirectional
FibreKor	Jeneric/Pentron	Glass	Unidirectional

Fig 2-4 *Scanning electron micrographs of glass-reinforced thermoplastics showing the degree of wetting of the fibers by the matrix.*

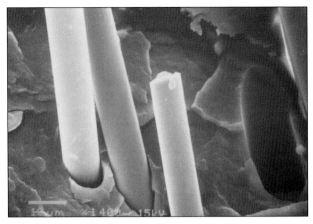

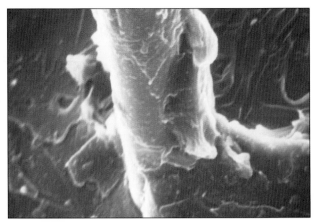

Fig 2-4a Poor wetting, resulting in weaker mechanical properties.

Fig 2-4b Effective wetting and coupling. Failure occurred away from the fiber-matrix interface.

are pre-impregnated with resin by the manufacturer or resination is required by the dentist or laboratory technician. Dental manufacturers use only standard industrial fibers; however, there is wide variation between products in fiber surface treatments, methods for incorporating the fibers into the polymeric resin, and chairside and laboratory processing methods.

History of Fiber Reinforcement in Dentistry

The first attempts to use fiber reinforcement in clinical dentistry began more than 35 years ago. In the 1960s and 1970s, investigators sought to reinforce standard polymethyl methacrylate dentures with glass[34] or carbon fibers.[26,33] In the 1980s, similar attempts were repeated,[5,16] and initial efforts were made to fabricate fiber-reinforced prosthodontic frameworks for implants,[4,8,31] fixed prosthodontic restorations,[25] orthodontic retainers,[6,27] and splints.[24] While these materials and techniques demonstrated improved mechanical properties, they failed to achieve general clinical acceptance because of insufficient enhancement of properties and awkward clinical manipulating procedures. Most of the proposed procedures involved intuitive manual placement of fibers into dental resins that were otherwise processed with routine methods. This approach was cumbersome since free fibers are difficult to handle and great care must be taken to avoid either damaging or contaminating them. Furthermore, while the addition of fibers increased mechanical properties, the degree of improvement was far below that achieved in other commercial applications. There were two reasons for the lower-than-expected mechanical results. First, the actual amount of fiber incorporated into the dental resins was low, typically less than 15% by volume. (Industrial products may contain 50% or even as much as 70% fiber by volume.) Second, the fiber reinforcement was not as effective as in theory because poor wetting of the fiber bundles by the resin led to insufficient coupling or even gaps between the fibers and resin[17] (Fig 2-4a). During testing, effective coupling usually results in failure not at the fiber-matrix interface but within the matrix[17] (Fig 2-4b).

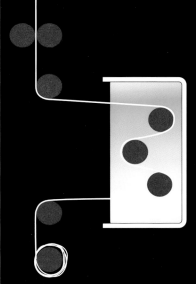

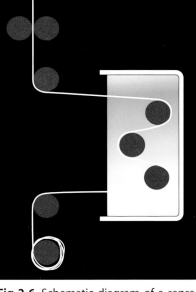

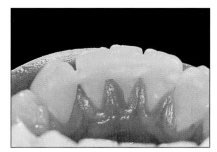

Fig 2-5 Manual application of a low-viscosity resin to a woven fiber product (GlasSpan, GlasSpan).

Fig 2-6 Schematic diagram of a representative manufacturing process for fabrication of pre-impregnated FRC. Fibers are pulled along a convoluted path through the resin bath. Pressure at the rollers forces resin into the fabric or fiber bundles.

Fig 2-7 Glass fiber–reinforced polycarbonate orthodontic retainer. (Courtesy of A. Patel and C. Burstone.)

In the late 1980s, dental researchers recognized the importance of effective coupling and complete impregnation of the fiber bundles by the resin and began to develop methods appropriate for dentistry. Since then two approaches have evolved. In the first, the dentist or laboratory technician manually applies a low-viscosity resin to the fiber bundles (Fig 2-5). While it provides complete wetting, this approach can be cumbersome and requires an additional step in the procedure. It does, however, offer versatility in the selection of fibers and resin. The alternate approach is to use fiber bundles that have been pre-impregnated during a controlled manufacturing process.[13] Although many different manufacturing methods are available, most involve pulling the fiber bundles through a convoluted path that forces the resin into the fiber bundles (Fig 2-6). As might be imagined, numerous manufacturing parameters control the final fiber dimensions and content, including the viscosity of the resin, speed of the process, tension on the fiber bundles, and so forth. These complex process parameters allow for high fiber content, complete wetting, minimum void content, and control of the cross-sectional dimensions in pre-impregnated FRCs.

Some of the earliest of these experimental pre-impregnated FRCs designed for dental applications were based on glass-reinforced thermoplastics.[14] Clinical trials were conducted using glass-reinforced polycarbonate as orthodontic retainers[28] (Fig 2-7). The esthetic retainers functioned satisfactorily and had a mean service life of 20.4 months. Most importantly, only 6% of those that failed were due to frank mechanical breakage of the fiber composites, confirming that the physical properties of these materials are adequate for this clinical application. Most of the clinical failures were the result of debonding of the retainers from the tooth surface.

A subsequent clinical trial evaluated the use of pre-impregnated glass-reinforced polycarbonate as the framework for acid-etched fixed partial dentures (FPDs).[2] Fourteen 3-unit restorations were placed both in anterior and posterior locations using adhesive techniques only and no tooth preparation. After 9 years, 3 restorations were still in service. All 11 failures were associated with separation in the region of the tooth-restoration interface; none was caused by frank mechanical breakage of the fiber-reinforced framework. The clinical failures occurred at the adhesive-tooth interface, the adhesive–fiber composite interface, or within the outer matrix of the fiber-reinforced composite. This study confirmed the adequate mechanical properties of FRCs for use in prosthodontic applications; however, it also demonstrated that the thermoplastic resin matrix is difficult to manipulate and offers poor bonding to tooth structures. These problems were resolved by switching to a bisphenol glycidyl methacrylate (bis-GMA)–based resin as the matrix for the FRCs.[11,19]

Four-year clinical trials of carbon fiber–reinforced polymethyl methacrylate implant-supported prostheses also demonstrated the potential for prosthodontic applications.[3] After 4 years, only 5 (19%) of 27 original prostheses had fractured; however, these experimental materials had less than half the strength of the commercial materials currently used.[8,31] Researchers recognized the potential for fiber-reinforced frameworks, but acknowledged the need for improved materials. Recent laboratory studies of provisional restorations have demonstrated that proper reinforcement with woven polyethylene fiber[32] or glass fiber[40] improves fracture resistance.

Continued research on glass-reinforced bis-GMA systems, combined with important manufacturer-designed fiber impregnation and packaging systems, has led to the commercial pre-impregnated systems available today: Sculpture/FibreKor, Splint-It (Jeneric/Pentron); and Targis/Vectris (Ivoclar). In both systems, the

fiber-reinforced strips typically measure several millimeters in cross section and several centimeters in length and are packaged in separately sealed, light-tight containers (Fig 2-8).

Using either pre-impregnated or hand-impregnated strips, a dentist or technician forms and fabricates the desired restoration, splint, or appliance, which is then cured. For most of the FRC procedures, a direct or indirect method can be used. Splints are commonly fabricated with a direct approach and light-cured, while fixed prostheses are typically fabricated by dental laboratories to minimize chair time and to allow for optimum esthetic and mechanical results. Both hand-impregnated and pre-impregnated systems are commercially available to the laboratory, although the latter are more widely used. Two commercial pre-impregnated systems are available for dental laboratories. Both use fiber composites to fabricate the framework, and the final tooth shape is then built with particulate-reinforced restorative composite. One system, Sculpture/FibreKor (Jeneric/Pentron), uses hand fabrication to form the framework and condense the strips (Fig 2-9). The other system, Targis/Vectris (Ivoclar), uses custom-made matrices (Fig 2-10a) and special equipment (Fig 2-10b) to apply pressure to the fiber strips during fabrication. In both systems, the main goals in the fabrication of the framework are to incorporate a sufficient amount of fiber reinforcement, minimize voids, and ensure strong bonding between both the layers of pre-impregnated fiber strips and the fiber framework and restorative composite. Clinical trials of the commercial systems, now in their third year, demonstrate satisfactory performance when appropriate designs, fiber volume, and manipulative procedures are followed, although a loss of surface luster was often observed soon after placement.[12] Some early designs of fiber-reinforced FPDs required replacement of the facings, but repair methods have been described to minimize the need to replace the complete restoration.[29]

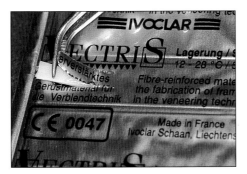

Fig 2-8 Pre-impregnated FRC strip being removed from its light-tight package.

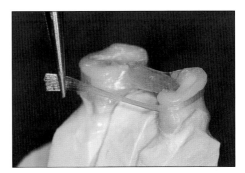

Fig 2-9 Fabrication of an FRC framework for a 3-unit FPD using the Sculpture/FibreKor system (Jeneric/Pentron).

Fig 2-10 *Fabrication of an FRC framework for a 3-unit FPD using the Targis/Vectris system (Ivoclar).*

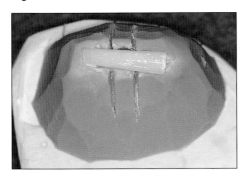

Fig 2-10a Custom matrix for maintaining shape.

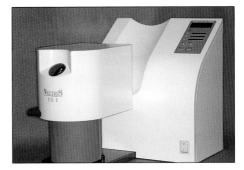

Fig 2-10b Equipment for applying pressure during curing.

Mechanics of Fiber Composites

Compared to traditional dental materials, the properties and mechanics of fiber composites are complex. While dental alloys are uniform, homogeneous, and isotropic—that is, they have the same properties regardless of the direction in which they are tested—fiber composites are heterogeneous and anisotropic, meaning their properties depend strongly on the direction in which they are tested relative to their fiber orientation. For unidirectional fiber composites, in which fibers run parallel and in one direction, properties are highest in the direction parallel to the fibers and lowest in the direction perpendicular to the fibers (Fig 2-11). As a result, restoration and appliance designs seek to place the reinforcing fibers parallel to the highest stresses. For example, in the pontic regions of fixed prostheses, the bulk of the fibers is placed in the mesiodistal direction, with fewer additional fibers placed at other orientations (Fig 2-12). Locations sustaining more complex forces, such as abutments and single crowns, require multidirectional fiber designs. Multiple fiber orientations can be achieved in one of two ways: either by placing unidirectional fibers in multiple directions, or by using a braided or woven fabric (see Fig 2-2). The availability of various fiber architectures, properties, and contents allows for a wide range of mechanical and handling characteristics in FRCs. An understanding of these mechanics helps one to understand the various products and their uses. A complete description of the mechanics of fiber composites can be found elsewhere[1,21]; however, the following brief discussion may be helpful.

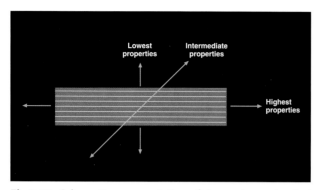

Fig 2-11 Schematic representation of change in mechanical properties related to fiber orientation in a unidirectional FRC.

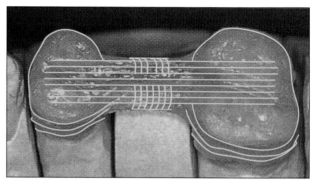

Fig 2-12 Schematic diagram of an FRC framework for an FPD. The majority of fiber is oriented in a mesiodistal direction, and the remaining fibers are at other orientations.

Rule of Mixtures

In prosthodontic applications, the two most important mechanical properties for FRCs are strength and stiffness. Stiffness or rigidity of the material is referred to as the modulus of elasticity. A high modulus is necessary for fiber-reinforced FPD frameworks because they must support the more brittle overlying restorative composite. This situation is analogous to metal frameworks supporting porcelain in a metal-ceramic prosthesis. In an ideal unidirectional FRC, the modulus as well as the strength in the fiber direction is proportional to the volume and individual properties of the fiber and the matrix. This relationship is known as the "rule of mixtures."[1] Because the properties of the fiber are usually much greater than those of the matrix, the rigidity and strength of a unidirectional fiber composite are largely dependent on the properties and volume of the fiber. Therefore, when the highest mechanical properties are desired in a single direction, as in a post or in the pontic region of an FPD framework, large volumes of high-strength unidirectional fibers are desirable. Where esthetics may not be critical, carbon fibers may be used. Where translucency is required in combination with good mechanical properties, glass fibers are generally preferred. Because of the necessity of having all fibers fully wetted by the resin, fiber volumes are generally limited to less than 50%. Typical pre-impregnated unidirectional dental fiber composites incorporating approximately 45% glass fibers have a flexure modulus in the range of 28 to 34 GPa and flexure strengths of about 600 to 1,000 MPa. These values are about 10 times greater than those for dental resin alone, and they represent the primary mechanical benefit of using fiber reinforcement in dentistry.

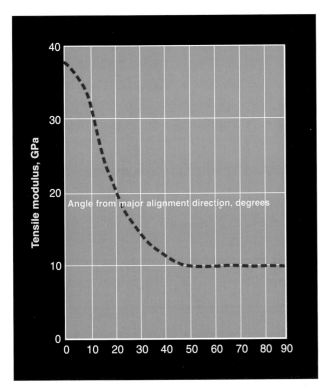

Fig 2-13 Effect of testing orientation on the tensile modulus of glass fiber–reinforced composite.

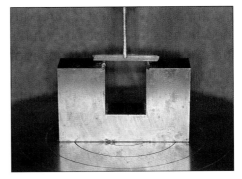

Fig 2-14 Flexure testing of an FRC sample.

When the direction of the force is no longer parallel to that of the fibers, the mechanical properties of the unidirectional composite decrease and become more dependent on the resin matrix. This correlated decrease in properties according to fiber direction follows an S-shaped curve[18] (Fig 2-13). Based on fiber volume, constituent properties (see Table 2-1), and effect of fiber orientation, the measured modulus values for the most common dental fiber products are reasonably consistent with the "rule of mixtures" predictions.[15] These types of relationships are used by dental researchers to design fiber composite materials and procedures for various clinical applications.

In addition to their mechanical properties, the handling characteristics of FRCs are also important, particularly for products handled chairside by the dentist. Fiber-reinforced composites have been used routinely as splints,[9,35,36] an ap-

plication for which ease of adaptation is critical to clinical success. Braided or woven fiber products such as GlasSpan (GlasSpan) and Splint-It (Jeneric/Pentron) readily adapt to misaligned and rotated teeth because of their fiber architecture. Woven polyethylene fiber products such as Ribbond (Ribbond) and Splint-It (Jeneric/Pentron) are even more manageable because of their fiber architecture and the low modulus of the fiber in compression.

Flexure Strength

In dental applications such as fixed prostheses, splints, and posts, FRCs are usually subjected to flexure or bending in clinical service. Accordingly, these materials are often tested in flexure in the laboratory (Fig 2-14), although the mode of failure and many other properties affect clinical performance. In particular, many investigators emphasize the importance of fatigue[38] and fracture toughness in predicting clinical performance of several classes of dental materials,[22] including fiber composites.[30] While clinical performance is the final determinant of success, flexure is still the most widely reported mechanical property, and test results are useful in developing and selecting new materials for clinical use and in comparing products. Furthermore, comparisons of flexure strength values obtained using similar test procedures can demonstrate improvement in categories of materials over time.

The experimental fiber-reinforced denture resins of the 1960s had properties only marginally superior to those of the resins themselves, and some reports even showed decreased strength with reinforcement due to poor adhesion between the fibers and the matrix.[16] As fiber contents were increased and the overall quality of dental fiber composites improved, their flexure strengths became sufficient for applications such as frameworks for fixed prostheses. The early thermoplastic-based dental fiber composites had flexure strengths of 200 to 500 MPa.[14] The earliest prosthodontic framework fiber composites, used on implant-supported prostheses, approached flexure strength values of approximately 250 MPa.[8,31] Contemporary methods for glass-fiber reinforcement of denture resins produce strengths of 265 MPa,[37,39] and reinforcement of dental resins with high-strength polyethylene fibers can achieve values of approximately 200 MPa.[23]

It is important to note that test methods, procedures for preparing the samples, and, in particular, the geometry of the test specimens all affect the calculated flexure strength. For this reason, care must be taken in comparing the results of different studies. A common sample geometry for flexure testing is a rectangular bar of 2 mm × 2 mm × 20 mm; however 2-mm × 1-mm × 20-mm samples are also used. The ratio of the length to the depth of the sample can affect measured flexure properties by as much as 80%.[20] Typical flexure strength values for commercial laboratory–processed fiber-reinforced composites range from approximately 300 to 1,000 MPa, depending on the specimen preparation and geometry.[7,10] The strength of prosthodontic metal alloys is usually measured not in flexure but in tension, but for purposes of comparison, the yield and ultimate strength of gold alloys typically are 500 and 750 MPa, respectively. Values for base metal alloys vary widely, but corresponding representative values are 600 and 1,100 MPa, respectively.

Mechanical Properties of Commercial Products

At this time, various formulations of FRCs are being introduced for a range of dental applications. Many properties and characteristics need to be considered in selecting an appropriate product for clinical use, including ease of handling, retention, esthetics, and clinical experience. However, mechanical properties are of particular importance because of the mechanical demands placed on these products in service. Table 2-3 summarizes the flexural properties of representative FRC products. The fiber type and architecture of these products are described in Table 2-2.

As noted above, a high modulus is important in prosthodontic frameworks, especially in the pontic region, because the fiber composite resists bending and supports the more brittle particulate-composite veneer. The combination of a high percentage of glass fibers and a unidirectional architecture provides a relatively high modulus and strength to this category of products while maintaining translucency, which gives the prostheses excellent esthetics. Careful manipulation, special equipment avail-

Table 2-3 | Flexural properties of fiber-reinforced composite products

Clinical applications	Product	Company	Flexure modulus (GPa)	Flexure strength (MPa)	
				Elastic limit	Ultimate
Laboratory-fabricated prostheses	FibreKor	Jeneric/Pentron	28.3	471	539
	Vectris-Pontic	Ivoclar	28.9	516	614
Laboratory- or chairside-fabricated prostheses	Connect	Kerr	8.3	50	222
	GlasSpan	GlasSpan	13.9	266	321
	Ribbond	Ribbond	3.9	56	206
	Splint-It				
	Woven	Jeneric/Pentron	9.2	170	220
	Unidirectional	Jeneric/Pentron	26.3	469	617
Posts	FibreKor	Jeneric/Pentron	25.0	—	920
	C-Post	Bisco	18.0	—	1,600

able in dental laboratories, and high-temperature curing impart strong mechanical properties to these products.

Products that can be used either in the dental laboratory or at chairside have a range of flexural properties because of the various types and orientations of the fibers employed in this category. These products offer a range of uses, including splints, retainers, posts, and chairside FPDs. Products with lower properties often have other benefits, such as ease of adaptability, which can be helpful in certain situations such as placing a splint on misaligned teeth.

Table 2-3 lists two flexure strengths: the value at the elastic limit and the ultimate value. The former occurs when the prosthesis' deformation is no longer reversible; beyond this value, permanent deformation of the prosthesis occurs. This is a clinically important value for fiber composites because it is often the point at which failure initiates even if it is not detectable visually. The ultimate flexure strength is the value at final failure. This value is obtained with standard testing procedures and is commonly reported in the literature.

References

1. Agarwal BD, Broutman LJ. Analysis and Performance of Fiber Composites. New York: John Wiley & Sons, 1980.

2. Altieri J, Burstone CJ, Goldberg AJ, Patel A. Longitudinal clinical evaluation of fiber-reinforced composite fixed partial dentures: A pilot study. J Prosthet Dent 1994; 71:16–22.

3. Bergendal T, Ekstrand K, Karlsson U. Evaluation of implant-supported carbon/graphite fiber-reinforced poly (methyl methacrylate) prostheses. Clin Oral Implants Res 1995;6:246–253.

4. Bjork N, Ekstrand K, Ruyter IE. Implant-fixed dental bridges from carbon/graphite reinforced poly(methyl methacrylate). Biomaterials 1986;7:73–75.

5. DeBoer J, Vermilyea SG, Brady RE. The effect of carbon fiber orientation on the fatigue resistance and bending properties of two denture resins. J Prosthet Dent 1984;51:119–121.

6. Diamond M. Resin fiberglass bonded retainer. J Clin Orthod 1987;21:182–183.

7. Dyer SR, Sorensen JA. Flexural strength and fracture toughness of fixed prosthodontic resin composites [abstract 434]. J Dent Res 1998;77:160.

8. Ekstrand K, Ruyter I, Wallendorf H. Carbon/graphite fiber reinforced poly(methyl methacrylate): Properties under dry and wet conditions. J Biomed Mater Res 1987; 21:1065–1080.

9. Freilich MA, Goldberg AJ. The use of a pre-impregnated, fiber-reinforced composite in the fabrication of a periodontal splint: A preliminary report. Pract Periodontics Aesthet Dent 1997;9:873–876.

10. Freilich MA, Karmaker AC, Burstone CJ, Goldberg AJ. Flexure strength of fiber-reinforced composites designed for prosthodontic application [abstract 999]. J Dent Res 1997;76:138.

11. Freilich MA, Karmaker AC, Burstone CJ, Goldberg AJ. Development and clinical applications of a light-polymerized fiber-reinforced composite. J Prosthet Dent 1998;80:311–318.

12. Freilich MA, Duncan JP, Meiers JC, Goldberg AJ. Clinical evaluation of fiber-reinforced fixed partial dentures: Preliminary data [abstract 2218]. J Dent Res 1999; 78:383.

13. Goldberg AJ, Burstone CJ. The use of continuous fiber reinforcement in dentistry. Dent Mater 1992;8:197–202.

14. Goldberg AJ, Burstone CJ, Hadjinikolau I, Jancar J. Screening of matrices and fibers for reinforced thermoplastics intended for dental applications. J Biomed Mater Res 1994;28:167–173.

15. Goldberg AJ, Freilich MA, Haser KA, Audi JH. Flexure properties and fiber architecture of commercial fiber-reinforced composites [abstract 967]. J Dent Res 1998; 77:226.

16. Grave AMH, Chandler HD, Wolfaardt JF. Denture base acrylic reinforced with high modulus fibre. Dent Mater 1985;1:185–187.

17. Jancar J, DiBenedetto AT. Fiber reinforced thermoplastic composites for dentistry. Part 1. Hydrolytic stability of the interface. J Mater Sci Mater Med 1993;4:555–561.

18. Kacir L, Narkis M, Ishai O. Oriented short glass fiber composites. III. Structure and mechanical properties of molded sheets. Polym Eng Sci 1977;17:234–241.

19. Karmaker AC, DiBenedetto AT, Goldberg AJ. Extent of conversion and its effect on the mechanical performance of Bis-GMA/PEGDMA-based resins and their composites with continuous glass fibers. J Mater Sci Mater Med 1997;8:369–374.

20. Karmaker AC, Freilich MA, Burstone CJ, Goldberg AJ, Prasad A. Performance of fiber-reinforced composites intended for prosthodontic frameworks [abstract]. Trans Soc Biomaterials 23rd Annual Meeting 1997:231.

21. Kaw AK. Mechanics of Composite Materials. Boca Raton: CRC Press, 1997.

22. Kelly JR. Perspectives on strength. Dent Mater 1995;11:103–110.

23. Ladizesky NH, Chow TW. The effect of interface adhesion, water immersion and anatomical notches on the mechanical properties of denture base resins reinforced with continuous high performance polyethylene fibres. Aust Dent J 1992;37:277–289.

24. Levenson MF. The use of a clear, pliable film to form a fiberglass-reinforced splint. J Am Dent Assoc 1986; 112:79–80.

25. Malquarti G, Berruet RG, Bois D. Prosthetic use of carbon fiber-reinforced epoxy resin for esthetic crowns and fixed partial dentures. J Prosthet Dent 1990;63:251–257.

26. Manley TR, Bowman AJ, Cook M. Denture bases reinforced with carbon fibers. Br Dent J 1979;146:25.

27. Mullarky RH. Aramid fiber reinforcement for acrylic appliances. J Clin Orthod 1985;19:655–658.

28. Patel A, Burstone CJ, Goldberg AJ. Clinical study of fiber-reinforced thermoplastic as orthodontic retainers [abstract 87]. J Dent Res 1992;71:526.

29. Rosentritt M, Behr M, Leibrock A, Handel G, Karl-Heinz F. Intraoral repair of fiber-reinforced composite fixed partial dentures. J Prosthet Dent 1998;79:393–398.

30. Rudo DN, Karbhari V. Physical behaviors of fiber reinforcement as applied to tooth stabilization. Dent Clin North Am 1999;43:7–35.

31. Ruyter IE, Ekstrand K, Bjork N. Development of carbon/graphite fiber reinforced poly(methyl methacrylate) suitable for implant-fixed dental bridges. Dent Mater 1986;2:6–9.

32. Samadzadeh A, Kugel G, Hurley E, Aboushala A. Fracture strengths of provisional restorations reinforced with plasma-treated woven polyethylene fibers. J Prosthet Dent 1997;78:447–450.

33. Schreiber CK. The clinical application of carbon fiber/polymer denture resin. Br Dent J 1974;137:21–22.

34. Smith DC. Recent developments and prospects in dental polymer. J Prosthet Dent 1962;12:1066.

35. Strassler HE, LoPresti J, Scherer W, Rudo D. Clinical evaluation of a woven polyethylene ribbon used for splinting. Esthet Dent Update 1995;6:80–84.

36. Strassler HE, Haeri A, Gultz JP. New-generation bonded reinforcing materials for anterior periodontal tooth stabilization and splinting. Dent Clin North Am 1999; 43:105–126.

37. Vallittu PK, Lassila VP, Lappalainen R. Transverse strength and fatigue of denture acrylic-glass fiber composite. Dent Mater 1994;10:116–121.

38. Vallittu PK. Comparison of the in vitro fatigue resistance of an acrylic resin removable partial denture reinforced with continuous glass fibers or metal wires. J Prosthodont 1996;5:115–121.

39. Vallittu PK. A review of fiber-reinforced denture base resins. J Prosthodont 1996;5:270–276.

40. Vallittu PK, Docent DT. The effect of glass fiber reinforcement on the fracture resistance of a provisional fixed partial denture. J Prosthet Dent 1998;79:125–130.

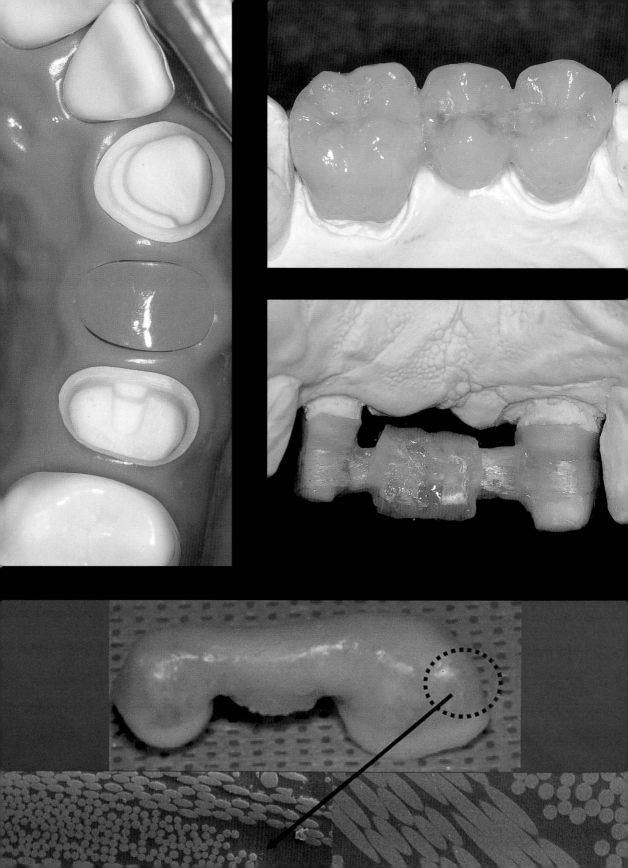

Laboratory-fabricated Tooth-supported Fixed Prostheses

Composition of an FRC Fixed Prosthesis

The fiber-reinforced composite (FRC) fixed prosthesis fabricated in the dental laboratory contains a substructure composed of bundles of glass fibers pre-impregnated with a resin matrix; covering this FRC substructure is a particulate composite. Figure 3-1 shows an FRC fixed prosthesis and its substructure. Mechanical testing and clinical experience have demonstrated that the FRC framework offers the strength and rigidity necessary to withstand the forces generated beneath the outer layer of particulate composite.[1,4,7,9,11,13,15] This two-component polymer prosthesis thus combines the best characteristics of both the fiber-reinforced composite (strength and rigidity) and the particulate composite (wear resistance and esthetics).[5,6]

Substructure and Framework

This chapter describes only the *pre-impregnated* FRC materials used for the construction of laboratory-fabricated prostheses. As explained in chapter 2, the pre-impregnated FRC is formed when the fibers and the resinous matrix are coupled together during the manufacturing process. This technique results in fibers that are uniformly pre-impregnated with matrix.[7,8] The cross section of a long fiber-reinforced composite bonded to a particulate composite is shown in Fig 3-2. Under three-point

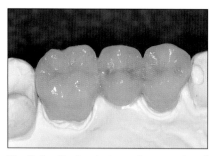 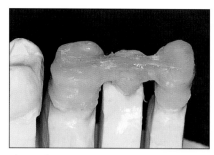 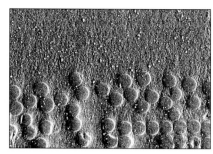

Fig 3-1a Occlusal view of a completed maxillary FRC 3-unit prosthesis.

Fig 3-1b FRC substructure for the prosthesis shown in Fig 3-1a.

Fig 3-2 Scanning electron micrograph cross section of a long FRC bonded to a layer of particulate composite.

loading conditions, pre-impregnated, unidirectional FRC has been proven capable of supporting 2 to 3 times the load of some woven FRCs that require hand impregnation, and it has exhibited up to 10 times the flexure modulus.[10]

The light- and heat-polymerized FRC materials used to make laboratory-fabricated prostheses have demonstrated up to 7 times the strength of particulate composite; moreover, these materials are much more rigid than those made of particulate composites.[3,4,14] Due to the translucent appearance of FRC materials, no additional masking material needs to be placed over the FRC substructure. This allows a relatively thin (approximately 0.5 mm) layer of particulate composite to be placed over the FRC substructure while maintaining an esthetic appearance.

Suprastructure and Veneer

Advances in particulate resin composite technology have enhanced and supplemented FRC technology. Some of the improved products—including Sculpture, Artglass Poly(mer)glass, Targis Ceromer, and belleGlass HP—employ new polymer formulations, improved filler particle distribution and loading, and intense light, vacuum, and heat polymerization. Together, these factors have improved the wear resistance and increased the elasticity of these improved composites, which in turn has resulted in increased impact and fracture resistance.[2,16–18] When used as the overlay or veneer, creating the anatomical shape and contour over the FRC framework, this new generation of composite materials provides the potential for a metal-free and ceramic-free prosthesis with long-term durability and service.

Materials

As noted in chapter 2, two commercial pre-impregnated FRC materials are currently available for use in fabricating fixed prostheses in the dental laboratory. Both of these systems, which are shown in Fig 3-3, use glass fiber composites to fabricate the framework; the final tooth contours are built with particulate-reinforced restorative composite. One system (Sculpture/FibreKor, Jeneric/Pentron) is a unidirectional glass material and employs *hand fabrication* to form the framework. The other system (Targis/Vectris, Ivoclar) is available in both unidirectional and woven glass forms and utilizes custom-made matrices and special equipment to apply light, heat, and pressure to the fiber strips during fabrication, resulting in an *equipment-fabricated* FRC framework.

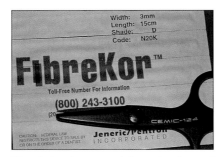

Fig 3-3a Commercial packaging of FibreKor (Jeneric/Pentron), a pre-impregnated long glass FRC material that employs a hand-fabricated technique.

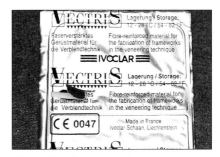

Fig 3-3b Commercial packaging of Vectris Pontic (Ivoclar), a pre-impregnated long glass FRC material that employs an equipment-fabricated technique.

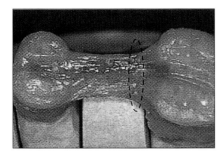

Fig 3-4a Hand-fabricated FRC (FibreKor) substructure highlighting the distal connector.

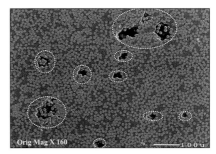

Fig 3-4b Scanning electron micrograph cross section of a FibreKor substructure in the connector region. Note the presence of small voids.

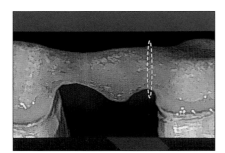

Fig 3-4c Equipment-fabricated FRC (Vectris) substructure highlighting the distal connector.

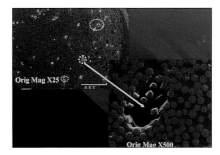

Fig 3-4d Scanning electron micrograph cross section of a Vectris substructure in the connector region. Note the presence of small voids.

The main goals in the fabrication of frameworks made with either system are to incorporate a sufficient amount of fiber reinforcement, to minimize voids, and to ensure strong bonding between the layers of pre-impregnated fiber strips and between the fiber framework and veneering composite. Figure 3-4 shows scanning electron microscope cross sections of hand-fabricated and equipment-fabricated FRC frameworks. Note that both systems exhibit a number of small voids in the connector areas. Such voids were found in all samples, independent of the system or material utilized. All of these study samples were made in one laboratory by careful, well-trained technicians. The number and size of the voids were minimized by the skilled efforts of these laboratory personnel. Prostheses made using the same techniques in the same laboratory have functioned satisfactorily in many different patients. It is likely that poorly made prostheses with large voids in critical areas would be less successful.

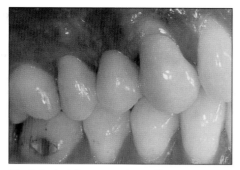

Fig 3-5 Facial aspect of maxillary FRC 3-unit prosthesis. The supragingival margin of the canine retainer blends easily with the non-prepared tooth structure apical to the finish line.

Table 3-1	Selection Criteria for Fiber-Reinforced Fixed Prostheses	
Indications	**Contraindications**	
Optimal esthetic result	Inability to maintain fluid control	
Metal free	Long span needed	
Decrease wear to opposing teeth	Patient with parafunctional habits	
Use of an adhesive luting technique	Opposing unglazed porcelain	

Clinical Applications for Extracoronal FRC Prostheses

There are several general indications for selecting a fiber-reinforced polymer prosthesis: *(1)* to attain an optimal esthetic result; *(2)* to deliver a metal-free prosthesis; *(3)* to decrease the potential for wear of the opposing dentition as compared to that of porcelain-veneered prostheses; and *(4)* to create the potential for bonding the prosthesis retainers to the abutment teeth.

These materials can be used anywhere esthetics is important, since the lack of metal or opaque materials allows for good translucency and a very natural-appearing prosthesis. This natural appearance at the cervical aspect of the prosthesis retainer also eliminates the need for the dentist to hide margins subgingivally, where they may cause periodontal problems for the patient. Supragingival margins blend in easily with the nonprepared tooth structure apical to the tooth preparation finish line, just as the overall prosthesis blends in with the ad-

jacent natural teeth (Fig 3-5). The resin composite luting materials that bond to the internal aspect of the polymer prosthesis retainers and to the dentin and enamel of the abutment teeth provide improved retention of the prosthesis. This feature may provide critical retention of a polymer prosthesis on abutment teeth that cannot be made to exhibit optimum geometric retention form.

Contraindications for selecting an FRC prosthesis include: *(1)* inability to maintain good fluid control, for example, in patients exhibiting chronic or acute gingival inflammation or when margins would be placed deeply into the sulcus; *(2)* a need for long-span prostheses, that is, those with two or more pontics; *(3)* patients who exhibit parafunctional habits; and *(4)* patients who have unglazed porcelain or removable partial denture frameworks that would oppose the prosthesis. Further, it should be noted that any resin composite surface exposed to oral fluids has potential for accelerated degradation in patients who abuse alcohol. Case selection criteria are summarized in Table 3-1. At this time there are no long-term clinical data regarding the overall success of the FRC prosthesis.

The use of adhesive cementation techniques requires maintenance of a contamination-free field. Rubber dam isolation is ideal and should be used where possible. At this time, FRC materials are not recommended for prostheses that replace more than two teeth, due to a lack of documentation regarding its ability to support greater edentulous spans and concerns regarding its flexure modulus, which is lower than that of metal alloys. In fact, Ivoclar recommends a maximum pontic span of 15 mm. A long-span prosthesis combined with lower flexure modulus can result in increased deflection of the framework and potential fracture of the relatively brittle composite veneer. Patients who brux or clench have an increased susceptibility to wear or fracture. Since clinical data are not yet available to substantiate how it would perform under these conditions, the FRC prosthesis should not be the treatment of choice until such data are available.

Clinical and Laboratory Procedures for Extracoronal FRC Prostheses

Tooth Preparations

Tooth preparations made for a reinforced polymer prosthesis constructed with either an equipment-fabricated system (Vectris, Ivoclar) or a hand-fabricated system (FibreKor, Jeneric/Pentron) must provide adequate space for the FRC substructure and the covering particulate composite. Clinicians should be aware of two specific abutment tooth preparation requirements: *(1)* the need to create an *adequate amount of tooth reduction,* and *(2)* the need to create a *marginal configuration* that permits an adequate amount of prosthetic material to be maintained at the margins of the retainers. Figure 3-6 shows optimal tooth preparations and the diamond burs used to make them.

Shoulder or chamfer preparations with minimally tapered axial walls and smooth, continuous finish lines (with a 90- to 120-degree cavosurface angle) are recommended. Additionally, at least 1.2 to 1.5 mm axial reduction on the facial and lingual surfaces and at least 1.5 mm occlusal reduction are required for adequate material thickness. (Ivoclar recommends at least 2 mm occlusal reduction if a nonadhesive cementation procedure is to be used to deliver the Targis/Vectris polymer prosthesis.) While these are the preparation guidelines advocated at present, no clinical or in vitro data are as yet available to indicate which type of finish line (the shoulder or heavy chamfer) is more desirable.

Experience has shown that the use of handfabricated FRC material (FibreKor) is optimized with the placement of a *proximal step* on axial walls adjacent to edentulous space, an *occlusal isthmus* on posterior abutment teeth, and a *lingual step* on anterior abutment preparations. Figure 3-7 shows these additional features. The proximal steps should be 2 to 3 mm wide and no more than 1 mm deep. They are prepared on the edentulous side of the coronal half of the axial walls of the abutment teeth. The isthmus, a shallow, 0.5 mm deep and 2 to 3 mm wide channel, is prepared on the occlusal surface of posterior abutment teeth. These features create additional room for the FRC substructure. The proximal box allows for sufficient material at the connector area and also gives the technician a positive stop for placing the pontic FRC support. The occlusal isthmus allows for a continuous "I-beam" configuration of FRC over each abutment tooth and across the edentulous space. A schematic of an ideal posterior full-coverage tooth preparation made for a FibreKor framework is shown in Fig 3-8a. Anterior tooth preparations for a FibreKor framework should exhibit a step or double-shoulder configuration on the lingual surface (Fig 3-8b) so that the laboratory technician can avoid creating a retainer with an overcontoured lingual axial surface.

Fig 3-6 *Tooth preparations made for extracoronal FRC prostheses and the diamond burs used to make them.*

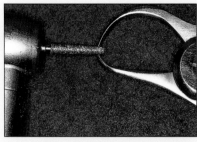

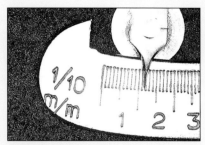

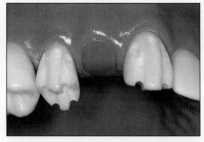

Figs 3-6a and 3-6b Round end-tapered diamond, measuring approximately 1.2 mm in diameter near the tip, which is used to make depth grooves.

Fig 3-6c Depth grooves made by placing the diamond bur completely into the tooth. Note the two-plane reduction on facial surfaces.

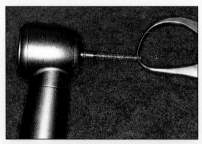

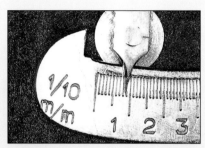

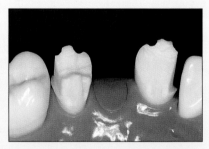

Figs 3-6d and 3-6e Round end-tapered diamond, measuring approximately 0.8 mm in diameter near the tip, which is used to "break" proximal contacts with adjacent teeth.

Fig 3-6f Broken proximal contacts.

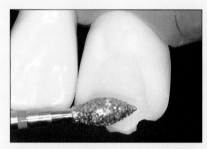

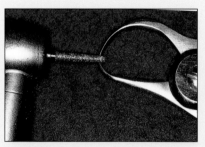

Fig 3-6g "Football"-shaped diamond, used on lingual surfaces to create lingual concavity in tooth preparation, thereby providing for adequate bulk of the prosthesis material and lingual concavity in the lingual surface of the retainer.

Figs 3-6h and 3-6i Round end-tapered diamond, measuring approximately 1.2 mm in diameter near the tip, which is used to complete the axial and occlusal tooth preparation.

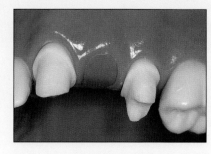

Fig 3-6j Tooth preparations, facial view.

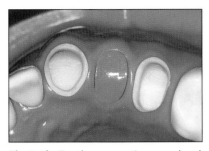

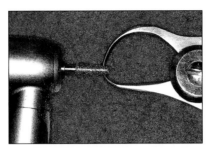

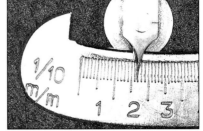

Fig 3-6k Tooth preparations, occlusal view. The depth of the preparation is the same (approximately 1.2 to 1.5 mm) on all aspects of the axial surfaces. Occlusal clearance should be 1.5 to 2 mm.

Figs 3-6l and 3-6m Fine grit, round, end-tapered diamond, measuring more than 1.5 mm in diameter near the tip, which is used to refine cavosurface finish lines of 90 to 120 degrees and round all line and point angles.

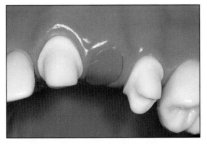

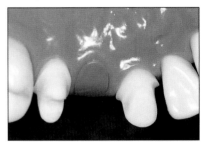

Fig 3-6n Final tooth preparation for extracoronal equipment-fabricated (Vectris) FRC prosthesis, viewed from the facial aspect.

Fig 3-6o Final tooth preparation for Vectris prosthesis, viewed from the lingual aspect.

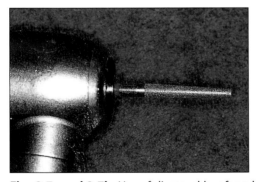

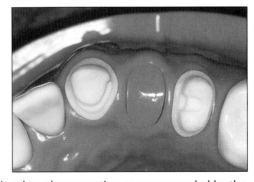

Figs 3-7a and 3-7b Use of diamond bur for additional tooth preparation as recommended by the authors for extracoronal, hand-fabricated (FibreKor) FRC prostheses. (See text for rationale and discussion.) (a) Fine grit, flat, end-tapered diamond, measuring approximately 1.0 mm, which is used to make additional preparation features in the FibreKor prosthesis. (b) Final tooth preparation for the FibreKor extracoronal prosthesis, viewed from the occlusal aspect. Note the proximal step and the occlusal isthmus on the posterior abutment tooth. Anterior abutment tooth preparation includes a step or double shoulder on the lingual and proximal surfaces adjacent to the edentulous ridge.

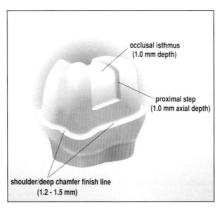

Fig 3-8a Schematic drawing of posterior abutment tooth preparation for the extracoronal FibreKor FRC prosthesis.

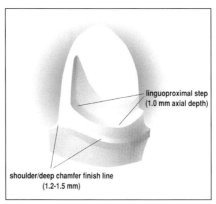

Fig 3-8b Schematic drawing of anterior abutment tooth preparation for the extracoronal FibreKor FRC prosthesis.

Working Casts and Dies

For both FRC systems, final impressions, dies, and working casts should be made using conventional methods and materials. An additional pour of the final impression is made so the dies of both abutment teeth can be left in one solid segment or cast for use while making the FRC substructure. The first pour of the impression is cut into individual dies, allowing the technician easy access to all retainer margins. A thin coating of a rubber separating material may be painted on the dies to within 1 mm of the finish line. An additional nonspaced separating material supplied by the manufacturer should then be placed over the remaining die surface.

Prosthesis Fabrication: Equipment-fabricated (Vectris) FRC Framework

It is important for the dentist to be familiar with the design features of an FRC prosthesis to fully appreciate tooth preparation requirements and to critically evaluate fiber-reinforced frameworks and fixed partial dentures (FPDs) made by the dental laboratory.

For the Vectris FRC framework, prosthesis fabrication involves three steps: *(1)* pontic bar fabrication with unidirectional FRC; *(2)* covering of the pontic bar and abutment dies with woven FRC; and *(3)* placement of particulate composite overlay. Figure 3-9 demonstrates the laboratory fabrication of an equipment-fabricated FRC prosthesis.

Framework fabrication begins with the placement of a wax wire at least 3 mm in diameter over and between the dies of the two abutment teeth. This wax pattern, which serves as the model for the pontic framework, should have adequate dimension in the connector area and should be slightly oval shaped. A silicone matrix covering the sides of the wax is made. The wax is removed, and the matrix is placed back over the dies on the working cast (Figs 3-9a to 3-9c). A sticky resinous substance (Vectris glue, Ivoclar) is placed at the occlusal and interproximal aspects of the abutment dies prior to placement of the FRC material.

The unidirectional FRC (Vectris Pontic) material (Fig 3-9d) is available from the manufacturer in the form of a bar that can be cut with special scissors to the desired length. At least two layers of this material are needed. The first layer is cut to the mesiodistal length of the edentulous space and placed into the matrix. The second layer is cut to cover the length of the occlusal surfaces as well as the edentulous space. This longer FRC layer is placed directly over the first layer. The cast is placed into the Vectris VS1 curing unit (Fig 3-9e), where the FRC is pressed (condensed and light polymerized) under vacuum. The polymerized FRC pontic is removed from the silicone matrix and trimmed with tungsten carbide burs. The gingival-occlusal thickness of the FRC covering the dies should be at least 0.3 mm and must cover at least three fourths of the occlusal surface. The finished pontic bar is air abraded with aluminum oxide at low pressure and then steam cleaned. Placement of the unidirectional FRC into the matrix, along with the untrimmed and then trimmed FRC pontic, is shown in Figs 3-9f to 3-9i.

Woven FRC (Vectris Frame) is used to cover the abutment dies and the previously polymerized pontic bar. In preparation for this, separator material is applied to the abutment dies and adjacent areas. All undercuts are blocked out with silicone putty material (Fig 3-9j). Vectris wetting agent (silane) is applied to the external pontic surfaces, and the excess is blown off after 60 seconds. The pontic bar may be held in place on the dies and within the silicone matrix with Vectris glue material. The woven Vectris Frame FRC is removed from its package, trimmed to size, and placed over the pontic bar (Fig 3-9k). The cast is again placed into the VS1 curing unit for light polymerization under vac-

uum (Figs 3-9l to 3-9o). The woven FRC is trimmed to within 1 to 2 mm of the abutment die finish line. The finished framework is air abraded with aluminum oxide and then steam cleaned. Vectris wetting agent is applied to all external surfaces of the finished framework, and the excess is blown off prior to placement of the particulate composite veneer material. Figures 3-9p to 3-9r show the FRC composition of different areas of the framework.

A modification of this technique is used if the prosthesis is to be cemented with a conventional, nonadhesive technique. In that case, the retainer component of the framework is made with additional thickness: woven Vectris Single is pressed and polymerized directly over the abutment dies before the pontic bar is made. Increasing the thickness of the framework increases its flexure modulus and rigidity.

Targis is the particulate composite veneer material used to create the outer layer of this FRC prosthesis. The Targis material is built incrementally using Targis Quick, a sensor-activated light-polymerizing unit (Fig 3-9s). This technique allows for the placement of a base color, dentin, incisal, and transparent materials, along with more intensive modifiers (Fig 3-9t). The completed 3-unit prosthesis is shown in Fig 3-9u. Following shaping and finishing, the prosthesis is placed into the Targis Power unit (Fig 3-9v) for the final application of light and heat to complete polymerization and maximize strength and other physical characteristics. Once this final polymerization is attained, the prosthesis is polished.

Fig 3-9 *Laboratory fabrication of an extracoronal equipment-fabricated (Vectris) FRC prosthesis.*

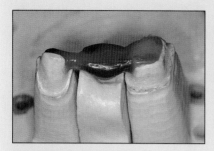

Fig 3-9a Final wax pattern for the pontic bar.

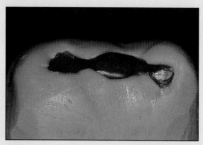

Fig 3-9b Occlusal view of the silicone matrix formed around the wax pattern.

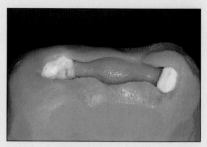

Fig 3-9c Silicone matrix after removal of the wax pattern.

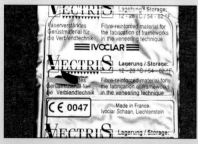

Fig 3-9d Unidirectional Vectris Pontic material being removed from its light-protected package.

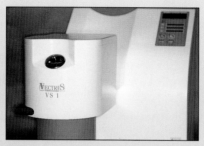

Fig 3-9e Vectris VS1 curing unit presses and light polymerizes the Vectris FRC material while under a vacuum.

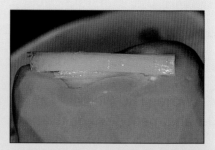

Fig 3-9f A minimum of two layers of Vectris Pontic material is placed into the silicone matrix. The first layer is cut to the mesiodistal length of the edentulous ridge, while the second layer is longer and extends over the occlusal surfaces of both abutment dies.

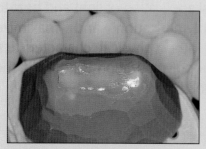

Fig 3-9g Polymerized Vectris Pontic within silicone matrix, prior to removal from the Vectris VS1 unit.

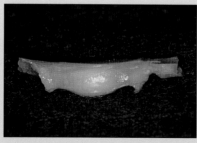

Fig 3-9h Polymerized Vectris Pontic upon removal from the silicone matrix.

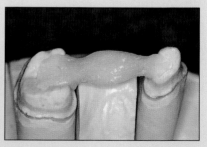

Fig 3-9i Trimmed Vectris Pontic placed back on abutment dies.

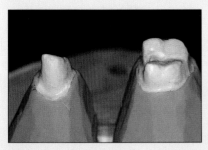

Fig 3-9j Undercuts apical to finish lines on abutment dies blocked out with silicone material.

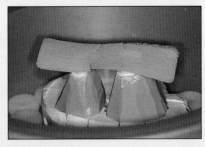

Fig 3-9k Woven glass Vectris Frame material cut to size and placed over the abutment dies.

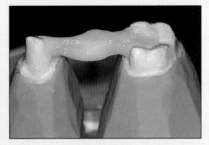

Fig 3-9l Polymerized and trimmed Vectris Pontic once again placed over the abutment dies prior to final placement and polymerization of Vectris Frame.

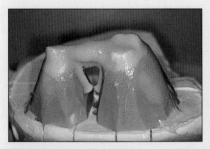

Fig 3-9m Combined Vectris Pontic and Vectris Frame immediately after polymerization but prior to removal from dies.

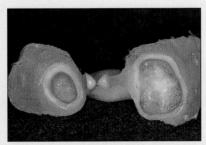

Fig 3-9n Undersurface of Vectris substructure after polymerization.

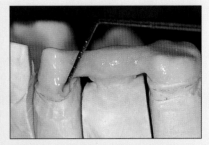

Fig 3-9o Completed Vectris substructure. An initial layer of particulate composite veneer is being added to the facial margin of the mesial retainer. Note the apicocoronal location of the pontic bar-coping interface, allowing space for the gingival embrasure in the completed prosthesis.

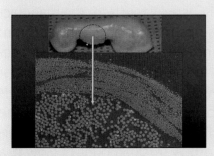

Fig 3-9p Scanning electron micrograph of the pontic, showing the variable architecture of FRC; woven material (Vectris Frame) external to the cross section of the long fibers (Vectris Pontic) is seen on the inside.

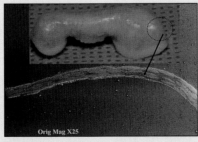

Fig 3-9q Scanning electron micrograph showing woven FRC at the distal retainer.

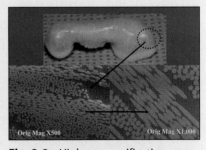

Fig 3-9r Higher-magnification scanning electron micrograph of the area shown in Fig 3-9q.

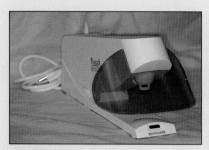

Fig 3-9s Targis Quick, a sensor-activated light-polymerizing unit.

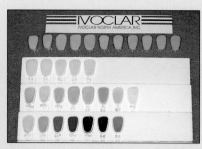

Fig 3-9t Some of the more intensive color modifiers available for the Targis particulate composite veneer used to create the outer layer of the FRC prosthesis.

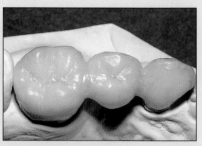

Fig 3-9u Completed 3-unit FRC (Targis/Vectris) prosthesis, viewed from the occlusal aspect.

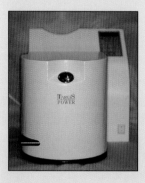

Fig 3-9v Targis Power, for the final application of light and heat, used after the prosthesis is completed to maximize polymerization.

Prosthesis Fabrication: Hand-fabricated (FibreKor) FRC Framework

For this material, prosthesis fabrication involves four steps: *(1)* coping fabrication; *(2)* pontic bar FRC connector placement; *(3)* fabrication of the FRC enveloping substructure; and *(4)* placement of the particulate composite overlay. Figure 3-10 demonstrates the laboratory fabrication of a hand-fabricated FRC prosthesis.

A thin "coping" of Opaceous body particulate composite (Sculpture, Jeneric/Pentron) is adapted to the dies (Fig 3-10a). The coping includes a cervical collar, which is placed on the axial wall to ensure that the FRC is contained above the cervical third of the axial walls during placement. A notch is also placed into each of the copings at the midproximal of the axial surfaces facing the edentulous area. This notch (Fig 3-10b), which corresponds to the proximal

step placed in the tooth preparation, will stabilize the FRC material when it is placed between the two copings. The copings are polymerized in the Cure-Lite Plus (Jeneric/Pentron) light box (Fig 3-10e). The completed copings are removed from the trimmed dies and placed on the second pour, solid die cast.

FibreKor FRC is available from the manufacturer in long strips measuring 3 mm or 6 mm wide and 0.3 mm thick that can be cut with ceramic scissors to the desired length. The wider strips are shown in Fig 3-10c. A bar of FRC is then formed by combining 5 to 7 strips of the 6-mm wide FRC cut to the appropriate interabutment length. A small amount of Flow It, a flowable composite supplied by the manufacturer, is placed into the notches of the copings to enhance the bonding between the oxygen-inhibited layer of the copings and the unpolymerized FRC. The connecting bar is then placed into the notches of the composite copings and condensed into a premade silicone matrix (Fig 3-10d). Use of the matrix provides a semi-rigid scaffold for condensing the FRC, thereby minimizing the number of voids incorporated into the bar. The working cast is again placed inside the Cure-Lite Plus light box to polymerize the FRC bar and bond it to the copings. The bar must be positioned to leave enough space between it and the opposing tooth, allowing for adequate thickness of external particulate composite while maintaining good gingival embrasure form. The polymerized FRC bar is shown in Fig 3-10f.

A long, single strip of 3-mm wide FRC is then bonded to one end of the polymerized pontic bar (Fig 3-10g). This strip is adapted and light polymerized continuously along the bar and around the axial surfaces of the copings. The Spectra-Lite 990 (Jeneric/Pentron), a hand-held light (Fig 3-10h), is used to polymerize this FRC strip in a stepwise fashion: only one segment at a time of the FRC strip is placed in the desired position and then selectively polymerized and bonded. When the entire strip has been adapted and bonded to the copings, the first portion of the substructure is completed. Alternatively, two strips of 3-mm wide FRC may be used in place of the single strip.

Additional strips of FRC are cut to size, placed, and bonded to the buccal, lingual, and cervical aspects of the FRC bar spanning the edentulous area. A continuous strip is bonded to the occlusal surface of one coping over the occlusal aspect of the FRC in the edentulous area and across to the occlusal aspect of the second coping. This stepwise construction of the FRC substructure results in the creation of a miniature pontic composed of bonded and light-polymerized layers of FRC, some of which are continuous with the FRC that was bonded to and around the abutment tooth copings.

An important characteristic of this fiber-reinforced polymer prosthesis framework is its "single-unit construction." While the framework is made in layers beginning with the opaque body particulate composite, all layers retain their oxygen-inhibited external surface prior to the placement of the composite layer. Since no modifications are made to the composite layers once they are polymerized, the integrity of the oxygen-inhibited layer is maintained and the potential for these layers to be contaminated with grindings, dust, grease, or debris is avoided. The goal of this approach is to create a unified prosthesis that lacks boundaries between layers, since these may serve as areas of potential weakness or separation within the fiber reinforcement. If boundaries are created, the substructure would have the potential to fail at *lower* loads than the component materials are ultimately able to withstand. The long fibers of the pontic area also encircle the axial walls or cover the occlusal surfaces of each of the abutment teeth. The completed FRC substructure is shown in Figs 3-10i and 3-10j. Figure 3-10k presents a cross section of the substructure of a retainer, showing the layer of FRC adjacent to the underlying opaque body particulate composite.

The FRC substructure features an oxygen-inhibited layer on its external surface that allows for the bonding of the outer layer of particulate composite Sculpture. This outer layer of composite is built incrementally, allowing for the placement of cervical colors, translucent coverings, and a variety of customizing options (Figs 3-10l and 3-10m). The completed 3-unit prosthesis is shown in Figs 3-10n and 3-10o. Following final light polymerization, shaping, finishing, and polishing, the prosthesis is placed in the Conquest Curing Unit (Jeneric/Pentron), a special oven (Fig 3-10p), at 110°C and in a 29-inch vacuum for 15 minutes to maximize its strength and other physical characteristics. Figure 3-11 shows the instruments used to shape, finish, and polish the fiber-reinforced FPD in the dental laboratory. Figure 3-12 shows an FRC framework for an anterior prosthesis.

Fig 3-10 *Laboratory fabrication of an extracoronal, hand-fabricated (FibreKor) prosthesis.*

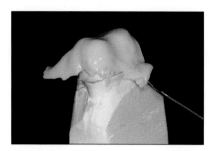

Fig 3-10a A thin coping of Opaceous body particulate composite adapted to the die.

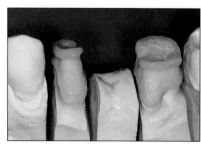

Fig 3-10b A completed, light-polymerized, opaque body particulate composite coping.

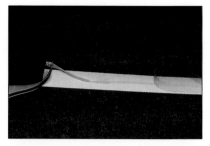

Fig 3-10c A single 6-mm wide strip of unidirectional, long glass FRC (FibreKor) being removed from its protective packaging.

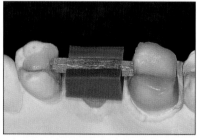

Fig 3-10d Sample of pontic bar created by placing and condensing 5 to 7 strips of 6-mm wide FibreKor into a prefabricated but cut-to-length silicone matrix.

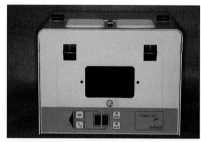

Fig 3-10e Cure-Lite Plus light box, used to polymerize the FRC bar and bond it to the copings.

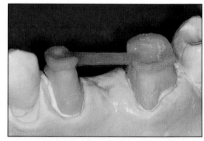

Fig 3-10f A polymerized pontic bar made of multiple layers of FRC spanning the edentulous region and bonding the abutment copings together.

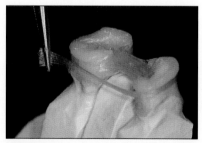

Fig 3-10g A continuous strip of FRC bonded to one end of the pontic bar and then wrapped around the axial surfaces of the copings while being polymerized segmentally.

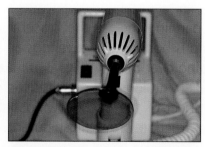

Fig 3-10h Hand-held Spectra-Lite 990 (Jeneric/Pentron) used to polymerize FRC while the strip of material is held in position during substructure fabrication.

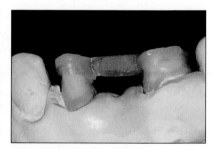

Fig 3-10i Facial view of the completed FibreKor FRC substructure. Note the apicocoronal location of the pontic bar–coping interface, leaving space for the gingival embrasure in the completed prosthesis.

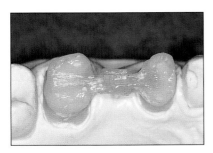

Fig 3-10j Occlusal view of the completed FibreKor FRC substructure.

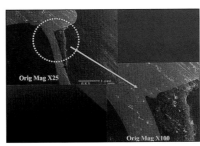

Fig 3-10k Scanning electron micrograph of an abutment coping cross section showing FRC *(right)* and particulate composite components *(left)*.

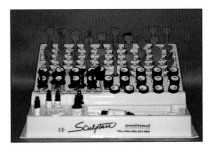

Fig 3-10l Sculpture (Jeneric/Pentron) particulate composite system used to place veneer over the FRC substructure.

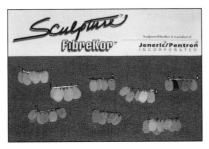

Fig 3-10m A variety of opaque body, dentin, and incisal shades, together with the color modifiers used in the Sculpture system.

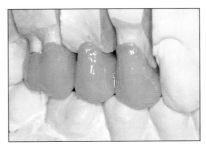

Fig 3-10n The completed maxillary posterior FRC 3-unit prosthesis, facial aspect.

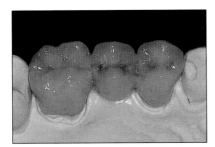

Fig 3-10o The completed maxillary posterior FRC 3-unit prosthesis, occlusal aspect.

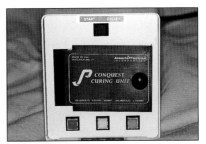

Fig 3-10p Conquest Curing Unit (Jeneric/Pentron), for the final application of heat under vacuum, used after the prosthesis is completed to maximize polymerization.

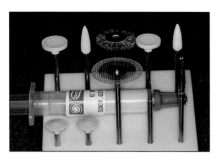

Fig 3-11 Instruments used to shape, finish, and polish the FRC prosthesis in the dental laboratory.

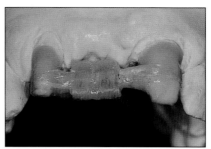

Fig 3-12a Example of an anterior hand-fabricated FibreKor FRC prosthesis substructure, facial aspect.

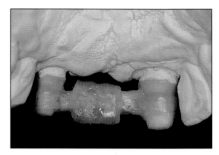

Fig 3-12b Hand-fabricated FibreKor FRC substructure, lingual view. *Note the bulk in the pontic region.* The pontic aspect of the substructure is a miniature model of the final pontic form.

Prosthesis Delivery

Materials required for the chairside delivery of an FRC prosthesis are as follows:

- High- and low-speed handpieces and burs
- Phosphoric acid gel etchant
- Fourth-generation (multiple bottle) or fifth-generation (single bottle) enamel-dentin bonding agent
- Dual-cured luting composite resin
- Visible light–curing unit

Figure 3-13 illustrates delivery of two maxillary anterior 3-unit FRC prostheses. As with delivery of any prosthesis, the dentist must check proximal contacts, occlusion, and anatomical form and shade, and make all necessary adjustments. Proximal contacts can be added by using a hybrid restorative composite after the surface has been roughened and by placing an unfilled resin on the overlay particulate composite. The shade of the prosthesis should be assessed using a manufacturer-supplied try-in water-soluble paste corresponding to the shade selected for luting. Minor adjustments can be made by selecting darker or lighter luting resins. The translucency of the FRC FPD allows the luting composite to play a role in the final shade.

Luting an FRC FPD involves the same procedures as for any bonded restorative procedure: isolation of the abutment teeth; treatment of the inner surface of the FRC FPD retainers; and treatment of the abutment teeth. First, the internal surfaces of the retainers are sandblasted with 50 μm aluminum oxide and then treated with a bonding agent supplied by the manufacturer. Concurrently, the abutment teeth are etched with 37% phosphoric acid, rinsed, lightly dried (not desiccated), and treated with a dentin bonding system (eg, Excite, Ivoclar or Bond It, Jeneric/Pentron). The sandblasted, primed FRC FPD is then delivered with a low-viscosity, dual-cured hybrid composite luting material (eg, Variolink II, Ivoclar or Lute-It, Jeneric/Pentron). This luting material will form a unified structure, linking the inside of the retainers to the etched enamel and hybridized dentin of the abutment teeth. The excellent esthetic result of this technique can be seen in Figs 3-13k to 3-13m. Note the close match of the shade and translucency to the natural teeth. For comparison, the patient's initial presentation with metal-ceramic crowns and prosthesis is shown in Fig 3-13n.

Figure 3-14 shows the adjusting, finishing, and polishing instruments used at chairside by the dentist prior to delivery. Both Ivoclar and Jeneric/Pentron supply finishing and polishing instruments that can be used for adjusting, polishing, and finishing FRC prostheses.

Fig 3-13 *Step-by-step procedure for delivery of two maxillary anterior FRC 3-unit prostheses.*

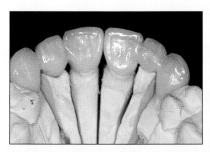

Fig 3-13a Lingual view of two completed maxillary FRC prostheses.

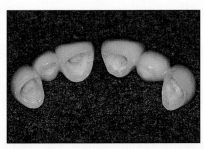

Fig 3-13b Internal aspects of FRC prostheses.

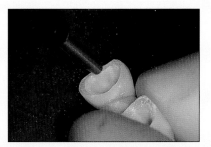

Fig 3-13c Internal surface of prosthesis retainer sandblasted with 50 μm aluminum oxide. Care must be taken since a continuous stream of air abrasion directed at the same location can perforate the retainer.

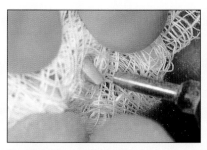

Fig 3-13d Air abrasion of metal cast core comprising a substantial portion of the abutment tooth.

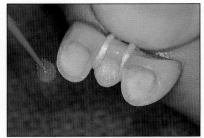

Fig 3-13e Internal aspects of prosthesis retainers coated with a thin layer of bonding agent-unfilled resin supplied by the manufacturer. Note the use of interproximal floss between the retainers and pontic. This provides a "handle" and greatly aids in the removal of luting material.

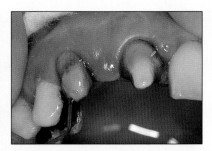

Fig 3-13f Abutment teeth treated with 37% phosphoric acid gel. Teeth are rinsed and lightly dried—not desiccated.

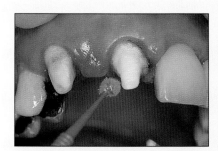

Fig 3-13g Placement of a fourth- (multiple bottle) or fifth- (single bottle) generation hydrophilic dentin primer-adhesive system.

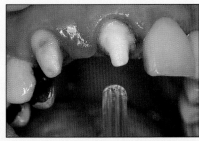

Fig 3-13h Excess primer-adhesive gently blown off abutment teeth.

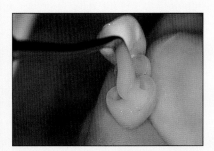

Fig 3-13i Low-viscosity, dual-cured hybrid composite luting material placed inside retainers.

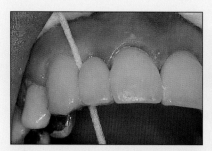

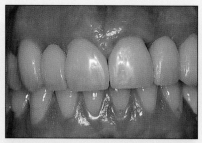

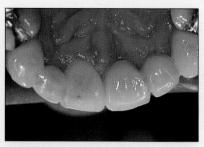

Fig 3-13j Excess luting material being removed quickly with interproximal floss and a composite sponge or small brush containing unfilled resin (primer-adhesive). Light polymerization is accomplished with a hand-held light source at the facial and lingual aspects of all abutment teeth for the manufacturer's recommended time.

Fig 3-13k Final result 1 week postinsertion, facial aspect. Note the close shade match and the natural translucency.

Fig 3-13l One week postinsertion, lingual aspect.

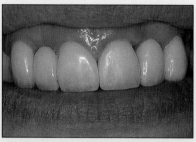

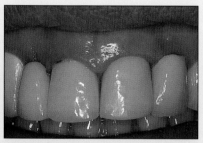

Fig 3-13m Relaxed smile, 1 week postinsertion. Note the importance of good esthetics at cervical areas of the prostheses.

Fig 3-13n Patient's initial presentation with metal ceramic crowns and a fixed prosthesis.

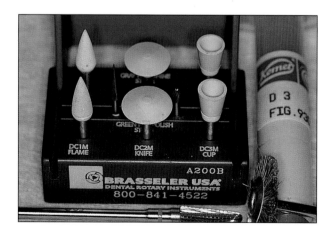

Fig 3-14 Instruments used to shape, finish, and polish the FRC prosthesis in the dental operatory.

Fig 3-15 *Intracoronal tooth preparations.*

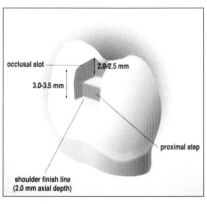

Fig 3-15a Schematic of an ideal tooth preparation design for a previously unrestored or minimally restored abutment tooth. Note the short proximal step.

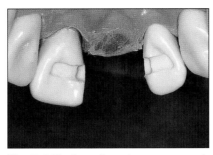

Fig 3-15b Anterior abutment tooth preparation.

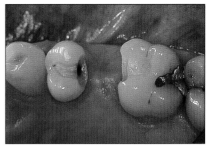

Fig 3-15c Posterior abutment tooth preparation.

Clinical Applications for Intracoronal FRC Prostheses

The FRC partial coverage fixed denture allows for a more conservative design when the abutment teeth are unrestored or have modest intracoronal restorations. When an implant is not an option, an etched metal (Maryland) bridge is the only other conservative fixed treatment alternative. However, these prostheses are becoming less desirable due to problems with debonding, graying of abutment teeth caused by metal showthrough, and overcontoured retainers. The advantages that apply for the complete coverage FRC prosthesis (esthetics, metal-free framework, porcelain-free veneer, and use of an adhesive cementation technique) also apply for the partial coverage FRC prosthesis.

Clinical and Laboratory Procedures for Intracoronal FRC Prostheses

Tooth Preparation

The preparation design can incorporate an existing cavity preparation as long as the walls are made to be divergent. Abutment teeth without restorations are prepared using a Class II composite inlay design with a short (occlusogingival) proximal step (Fig 3-15). A fully extended proximal box is unnecessary since the FRC cannot be placed apical to the contact area and at the same time maintain adequate embrasure form. Only particulate composite would be used to fill the portion of the box apical to the contact, and this would provide no benefit to the overall restoration. This point is clearly demonstrated in Fig 3-16h, where the existing restoration necessitated the box on the distal of the premolar. Observe the extent of the FRC pontic bar in relation to the contact area. The particulate composite apical to FRC does not add to the overall structural integrity of the prosthesis.

Fig 3-16 *Construction of an intracoronal FRC prosthesis substructure using hand-fabricated FibreKor FRC.*

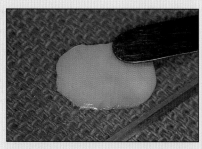

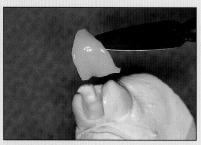

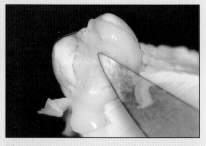

Fig 3-16a A thin layer of Opaceous body particulate composite, condensed on a glass tray.

Fig 3-16b A thin layer of Opaceous body composite being placed over the abutment die.

Fig 3-16c Opaceous body composite being adapted to the die.

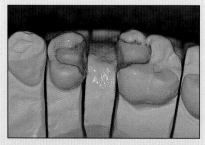

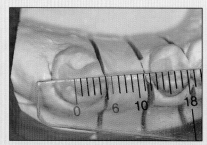

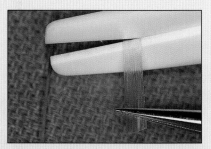

Fig 3-16d Unpolymerized Opaceous composite, extended to the finish lines of the tooth preparations, providing a sticky substrate for the addition of FRC.

Fig 3-16e Measurement of the length of the edentulous span and the distance covering the occlusal aspects of the preparations.

Fig 3-16f Multiple 6-mm wide FibreKor strips cut to size with ceramic scissors. Strips of two different sizes are needed: *(1)* 6 to 7 shorter-size strips to extend across the edentulous ridge between the axial walls of the two proximal steps; and *(2)* 2 to 3 longer-size strips to extend across the ridge covering the occlusal aspects (isthmus areas) of the preparations.

Laboratory Fabrication

The laboratory fabrication of an intracoronal prosthesis is shown in Fig 3-16. Dies and working casts should be fabricated in the same manner as for the complete coverage prosthesis. The intracoronal prosthesis can be made with either the equipment-fabricated or hand-

fabricated system; the latter system is illustrated in Fig 3-16. With the hand-fabricated FibreKor system, the framework design for an intracoronal prosthesis is less complicated than for a complete coverage prosthesis because it eliminates the need for circumferential wrapping of the FRC around the axial walls of the abutment teeth. A thin layer of Opaceous body particu-

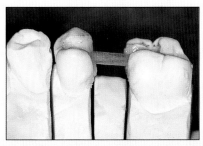

Fig 3-16g Pontic bar, made by placing and condensing the shorter strips into the silicone matrix (see Fig 3-10e).

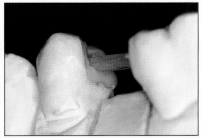

Fig 3-16h FRC pontic bar. The bar is not placed below the proximal contact area; thus, the proximal tooth preparation should not extend apical to the contact area unless a previous restoration or caries dictates continued apical tooth preparation.

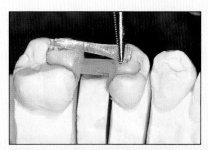

Fig 3-16i Placement of at least 2 of the longer FibreKor strips over the pontic bar and extended to cover the isthmus areas of the preparations.

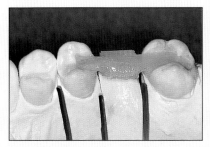

Fig 3-16j Completed intracoronal prosthesis substructure.

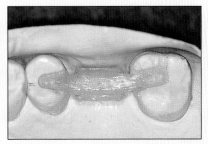

Fig 3-16k Completed substructure, occlusal aspect. Note the extension of FRC on the buccal and lingual aspects of the pontic. The FRC pontic should be a miniature model of the final pontic form to give adequate support for the 1.5- to 2.0-mm thickness of particulate composite veneer and to help prevent veneer fracture.

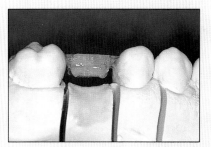

Fig 3-16l Facial view of completed substructure. Note that apicocoronal pontic bar placement will not interfere with final gingival embrasure form.

late composite is placed on the dies on the floor of the preparation and light polymerized (Figs 3-16a to 3-16d). Six or 7 FRC strips are cut to size and then placed over the opaque layer within each preparation and across the edentulous space (Figs 3-16e to 3-16g). The FRC is polymerized, and then an additional 12 to 15 strips of FRC are added to the buccal, lingual, and cervical aspects to create a miniature pontic shape (Figs 3-16j to 3-16l). The completed anatomic form of the pontic and retainers is developed with particulate composite. An equipment-fabricated Targis/Vectris intracoronal prosthesis designed to replace a mandibular molar is shown in Fig 3-17.

Fig 3-17 *Targis/Vectris intracoronal FRC prosthesis replacing a mandibular molar. (Courtesy of Dr Thomas Trinkner.)*

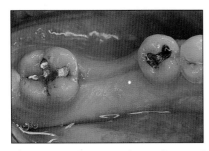

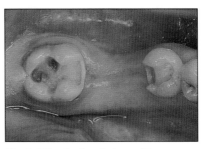

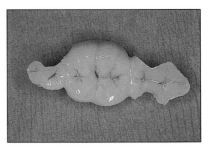

Fig 3-17a Preoperative view of mandibular posterior quadrant with minimally restored abutment teeth.

Fig 3-17b Occlusal view of intracoronal tooth preparations.

Fig 3-17c Completed Vectris intracoronal FRC prosthesis, occlusal view.

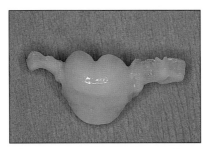

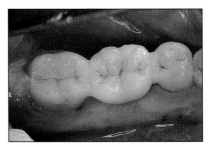

Fig 3-17d Vectris prosthesis, facial view.

Fig 3-17e Completed Vectris prosthesis postdelivery.

Prosthesis Delivery

Materials required for the chairside delivery of an intracoronal FRC prosthesis are as follows:

- Rubber dam
- High- and low-speed handpieces and burs
- Phosphoric acid gel etchant
- Fourth-generation (multiple bottle) or fifth-generation (single bottle) enamel-dentin bonding agent
- Dual-cure luting composite resin
- Visible light–curing unit

Figure 3-18 illustrates delivery of an intracoronal FRC prosthesis, beginning with verification of marginal fit, occlusion, and shade. Water-soluble shades of the luting composite may be used as recommended for complete coverage prostheses. After adjustments are made, the teeth should be isolated with a rubber dam. The abutments are then etched and coated with a dentin primer-adhesive. The inner aspects of the inlay retainers are lightly sandblasted with 50 μm aluminum oxide and then coated with primer-adhesive followed by a dual-cure luting composite. After light polymerization and removal of the rubber dam, occlusion is reconfirmed. Any final adjustments can be made with 30 fluted carbide finishing burs and paper disks. Rubber polishing points can be used for the final finish. The final esthetic result is shown in Fig 3-18h. A combination intracoronal-extracoronal FRC prosthesis and its framework is shown from a variety of views in Fig 3-19.

Fig 3-18 *Step-by-step procedure for delivery of an intracoronal FibreKor FRC 3-unit prosthesis.*

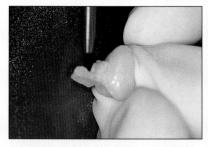

Fig 3-18a Internal aspects of prosthesis retainers carefully sandblasted with 50 µm aluminum oxide. Internal aspects of prosthesis retainers coated with a thin layer of bonding agent-unfilled resin supplied by the manufacturer.

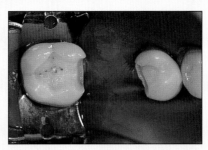

Fig 3-18b Final intracoronal abutment tooth preparations with rubber dam.

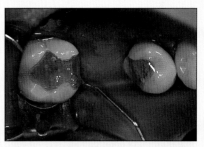

Fig 3-18c Abutment teeth treated with 37% phosphoric acid gel. Teeth are rinsed and lightly dried—not desiccated.

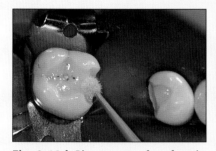

Fig 3-18d Placement of a fourth- (multiple bottle) or fifth- (single bottle) generation hydrophilic dentin primer-adhesive system. Excess primer-adhesive is gently blown off the abutment teeth.

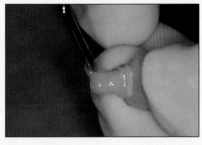

Fig 3-18e Low-viscosity, dual-cured hybrid composite luting material being placed inside the retainers.

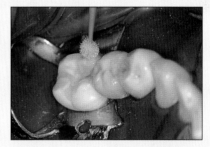

Fig 3-18f Excess luting material being removed quickly with a composite sponge containing unfilled resin (primer-adhesive). Light polymerization is accomplished with a hand-held light source at the facial and lingual aspects of all abutment teeth for the manufacturer's recommended time.

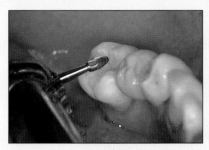

Fig 3-18g Final adjustment of the occlusion with multifluted carbide finishing burs. *Special note: occlusal adjustment should not be attempted until after delivery.* Fracture of retainers may occur if occlusion is adjusted prior to luting of the prosthesis to abutment teeth.

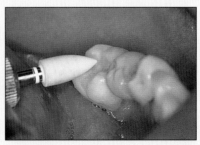

Fig 3-18h Final finishing with a rubber point.

Fig 3-19 Combination intracoronal-extracoronal FibreKor FRC prosthesis.

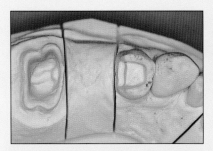

Fig 3-19a Occlusal view of the final tooth preparations on a working cast.

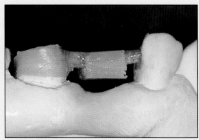

Fig 3-19b Facial view of the prosthesis substructure showing adequate bulk of the FRC in the pontic area and adequate room for gingival embrasures.

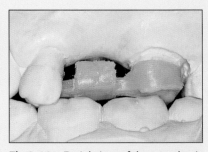

Fig 3-19c Facial view of the prosthesis substructure mounted to the opposing arch cast. Note the space available for occlusal veneer of the particulate composite.

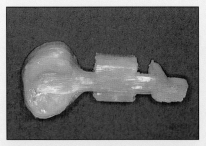

Fig 3-19d Occlusal view of the prosthesis substructure. Note the buccolingual bulk in the pontic area, providing good support for particulate composite veneer.

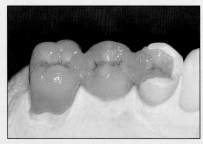

Fig 3-19e Completed intracoronal-extracoronal prosthesis on the working cast.

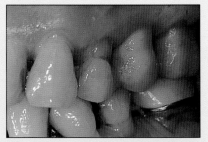

Fig 3-19f Completed intracoronal-extracoronal prosthesis in situ. Note the close match of the shade and translucency with the natural tooth structure of the premolar abutment.

Recommendations

Fiber-reinforced prostheses may prove to be a successful modality for fixed tooth replacement, providing many benefits to patients resulting from the natural esthetic appearance of a metal-free prosthesis and the inherent adhesive nature of polymer materials. The adhesive qualities may permit the use of abutment teeth that exhibit classic geometric retention and resistance form without the need for elective endodontics, surgical crown lengthening procedures, and, in some cases, the apical placement of finish lines.

Furthermore, favorable strength, esthetics, and adhesive properties make the intracoronal fiber-reinforced prosthesis uniquely well-suited for the minimally invasive replacement of a single missing tooth adjacent to unrestored or minimally restored abutment teeth. Multiyear clinical studies are currently in progress to determine the value and efficacy of the FRC prosthesis as a long-term tooth replacement.

References

1. Altieri JV, Burstone CJ, Goldberg AJ, Patel AP. Longitudinal clinical evaluation of fiber-reinforced composite fixed partial dentures: A pilot study. J Prosthet Dent 1994;71:16–22.

2. Fahl N, Casellini RC. Ceramor/FRC technology: The future of biofunctional adhesive aesthetic dentistry. Signature 1997;4(2):7–13.

3. Freilich MA, Karmaker AC, Burstone CJ, Goldberg AJ. Flexure strength of fiber-reinforced composites designed for prosthodontic application [abstract 999]. J Dent Res 1997;76(special issue):138.

4. Freilich MA, Karmaker AC, Burstone CJ, Goldberg AJ. Flexure strength and handling characteristics of fiber-reinforced composites used in prosthodontics [abstract 1361]. J Dent Res 1997;76:184.

5. Freilich MA, Duncan JP, Meiers JC, Goldberg AJ. Preimpregnated, fiber-reinforced prostheses. Part I. Basic rationale and complete-coverage and intracoronal fixed partial denture designs. Quintessence Int 1998;29:689–696.

6. Freilich MA, Karmaker AC, Burstone CJ, Goldberg AJ. Development and clinical applications of a light-polymerized fiber-reinforced composite. J Prosthet Dent 1998;80:311–318.

7. Freilich MA, Duncan JP, Meiers JC, Goldberg AJ. Clinical evaluation of fiber-reinforced fixed partial dentures: Preliminary data [abstract 2218]. J Dent Res 1999;78:383.

8. Goldberg AJ, Burstone CJ. The use of continuous fiber reinforcement in dentistry. Dent Mater 1992;8:197–202.

9. Goldberg AJ, Burstone CJ, Hadjinikolaou I, Jancar J. Screening of matrices and fibers for reinforced thermoplastics intended for dental applications. J Biomed Mater Res 1994;28:167–173.

10. Goldberg AJ, Freilich MA, Haser KA, Audi JH. Flexure properties and fiber architecture of commercial fiber reinforced composites [abstract 967]. J Dent Res 1998; 77:226..

11. Hadjinikolaou I, Goldberg AJ. Flexural behavior of clinically relevant fiber-reinforced composites [abstract 1190]. J Dent Res 1992;71:664.

12. Jancar J, DiBenedetto AT, Goldberg AJ. Thermoplastic fibre-reinforced composites for dentistry. Part II. Effect of moisture on flexural properties of unidirectional composites. J Mater Sci Mater Med 1993;4:562–568.

13. Karmaker AC, DiBenedetto AT, Goldberg AJ. Extent of conversion and its effect on the mechanical performance of Bis-GMA/PEGDMA based resins and their composites with continuous glass fibers. J Mater Sci Mater Med 1997;8:369–376.

14. Karmaker AC, DiBenedetto AT, Goldberg AJ. Fiber reinforced composite materials for dental appliances. Presented at Society of Plastic Engineers Annual Technical Conference, Indianapolis, 5-9 May 1996.

15. Patel A, Burstone CJ, Goldberg AJ. Clinical study of fiber-reinforced thermoplastic as orthodontic retainers [abstract 87]. J Dent Res 1992;71:526.

16. Radz GM, Nash RW, Leinfelder VF. An improved composite-onlay system. Compend Contin Educ Dent 1997;18(2):98,100–102,104.

17. Samadzadeh A, Bardwell D, Abdoushela A. Marginal adaptability of two different ceramic inlay systems in vitro [abstract 1434]. J Dent Res 1997;76(special issue):193.

18. Suzuki S, Suzuki SH, Kramer C. Enamel wear against resin composite and ceramic C&B materials [abstract 2454]. J Dent Res 1997;76(special issue):320.

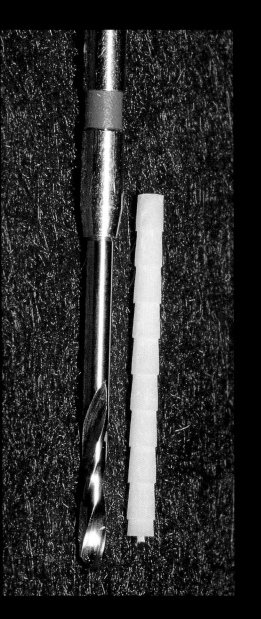

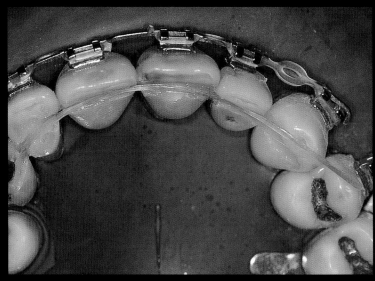

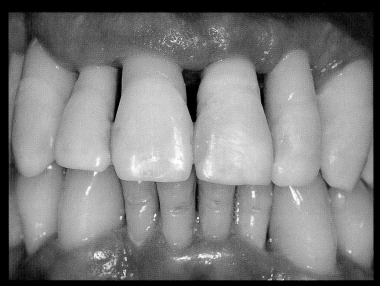

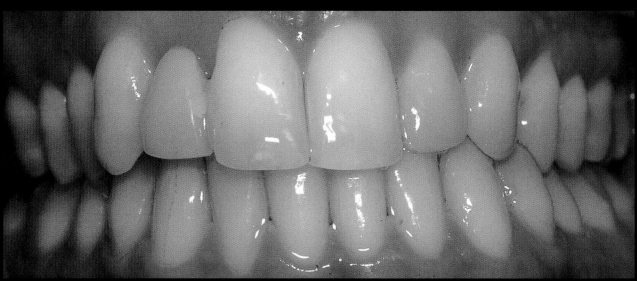

Chairside Applications of FRC

■ The properties of fiber-reinforced composites (FRCs) that make them well suited for various chairside applications include strength; desirable esthetic characteristics; ease of use; adaptability to various shapes; and potential for direct bonding to tooth structure. Among the many direct intraoral applications for this technology are splinting of mobile teeth, replacement of missing teeth, and fabrication of endodontic posts.

Tooth Stabilization and Splints

FRC materials are an excellent choice for the stabilization of hypermobile teeth. Chairside-fabricated fixed splints have previously been made from material combinations that have included resin composites,[21,23,28,34] wire,[3] wire mesh,[10,20,33] wire embedded in amalgam,[29,33] and resin and fiber mesh embedded in composite.[26,41] All of these materials suffered from various problems: poor handling characteristics, overbulking, insufficient bonding of the internal structural materials to the dental resins, and poor esthetic outcome.

FRC stabilization can be either intracoronal or extracoronal, depending on the clinical situation. The intracoronal technique requires a prepared horizontal channel that will accommodate the width and thickness of the FRC reinforcement material.[42,43] The dimensions of this channel usually range from 2.0 to 3.0 mm wide and from 1.0 to 2.0 mm deep. This channel is prepared in the middle to incisal third of the teeth. Mandibular

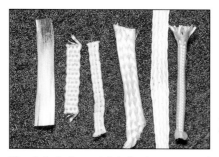

Fig 4-1 *(Left to right)* Pre-impregnated splint material (with the resin removed to show glass fibers): Splint-It unidirectional, Splint-It woven. Non–pre-impregnated polyethylene splint material: Ribbond, Connect. Non–pre-impregnated glass fibers: GlasSpan tape, GlasSpan rope.

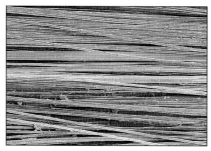

Fig 4-2 Scanning electron micrograph image of glass fibers (Splint-It unidirectional) with the resin removed. (Original magnification × 150.)

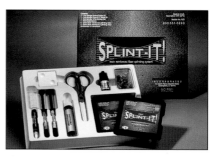

Fig 4-3 Commercially available pre-impregnated FRC splint material showing contents.

splints are usually placed on the lingual surfaces, while a maxillary splint can be placed on either the lingual or facial surface, depending on the occlusal relationships between the teeth.[43,46] The facial approach has the advantage of maintaining the occlusal stops on sound tooth structure, preventing the restorative (particulate) composite from interfering with function. Intracoronal splints for posterior teeth require channels that are usually placed on the occlusal surface; the channel can be prepared into an existing restoration and then inserted into particulate composite, which is placed within the channel preparation.

FRC materials are available with different fiber architectures, as described in chapter 2. Fiber architecture has a significant impact on both mechanical properties and handling characteristics. Woven fiber is less technique-sensitive and easier to manipulate because it has less memory than unidirectional fiber and is the best choice for rotated or malpositioned teeth. Unidirectional fiber has greater flexure strength and rigidity and is the better choice for high-stress situations.

Currently, two categories of fiber reinforcement material can be used for intraoral use: pre-impregnated and non–pre-impregnated (Fig 4-1).

Resin Pre-impregnated FRC Splinting Technique

Pre-impregnated material (Splint-It, Jeneric/Pentron) has two fiber designs: a 2-mm woven fiber and a 3-mm unidirectional fiber (Figs 4-2 and 4-3). The intracoronal approach can be seen in Fig 4-4; the extracoronal approach in Fig 4-5.

Materials required for the intraoral (chairside) fabrication of a periodontal splint are as follows:

- Diagnostic cast
- Rubber dam
- Wedges, Stimudents, high-viscosity polyvinyl siloxane impression material
- High-speed handpiece and burs
- Phosphoric acid gel etchant
- Fourth-generation (multiple bottle) or fifth-generation (single bottle) enamel-dentin bonding agent
- Intraoral FRC material (Splint-It, Jeneric/Pentron)
- Visible light–curing flowable particulate composite resin
- Visible light–curing unit

Fig 4-4 Intracoronal splinting technique using pre-impregnated FRC.

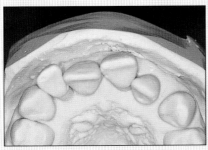

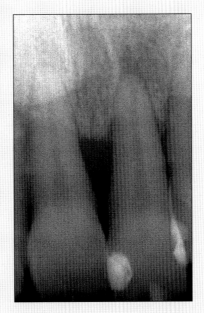

Fig 4-4a Diagnostic stone cast of patient at initial examination, used to plan the channel preparations and measure the length of FRC material.

Fig 4-4b Radiograph showing the extent of bone loss.

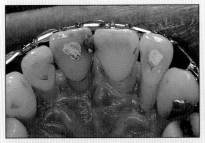

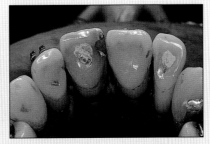

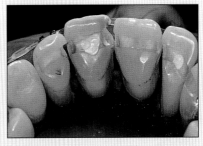

Fig 4-4c Maxillary teeth have been stabilized and put into proper arch contour by means of labial brackets and orthodontic wire ligation.

Fig 4-4d Rubber dam application following orthodontic wire removal and prior to slot preparation and FRC placement. The lingual/facial surfaces to be bonded are pumiced and interproximal surfaces are cleaned using interproximal finishing strips.

Fig 4-4e A lingual channel preparation, 2 mm wide and 2 mm deep, placed from canine to canine and including the proximal contact areas. In this clinical case, deficient Class III restorations were removed with the channel preparation. Wedges or high-viscosity polyvinyl siloxane impression material may be placed interproximally to limit the gingival-proximal extent of any excess resin.

Fig 4-4f After the channel and the interproximal surfaces are etched and rinsed, use of a fifth-generation (single bottle) or fourth-generation (multiple bottle) enamel-dentin bonding system. Small amounts of high-viscosity visible light–curing flowable particulate composite resin are added to the interproximal areas to act as a bridge between the teeth and the apical covering of the FRC material. Flowable particulate composite is placed into the prepared slots prior to the placement of the FRC splint material. The orthodontic stabilization is again in place to prevent movement of the teeth during the FRC insertion process.

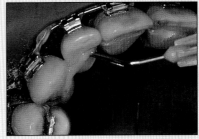

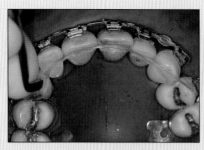

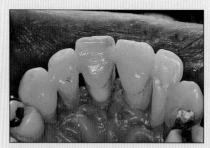

Fig 4-4g Two or three strips of unidirectional Splint-It material inserted into the particulate composite resin bed of the lingual channel and then light polymerized for 60 seconds per strip. A less viscous flowable or hybrid particulate composite is placed over these strips to fill the remainder of the depth of the channel to the level of the lingual surface.

Fig 4-4h Lingual view of finished FRC lingual slot splint with the orthodontic band-wire stabilization removed. The splint is contoured and finished as necessary and adjusted for occlusion.

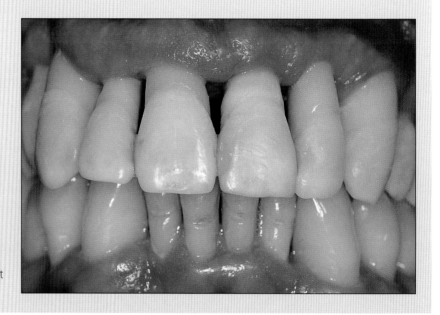

Fig 4-4i Facial view of FRC lingual slot splint. Note the excellent esthetic result.

Fig 4-5 *Extracoronal splinting technique using pre-impregnated FRC material.*

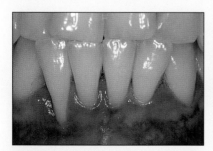

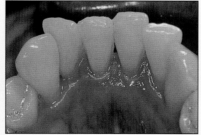

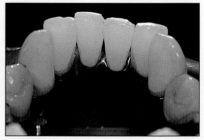

Fig 4-5a Facial view of mandibular teeth to be splinted.

Fig 4-5b Lingual view of mandibular teeth to be splinted.

Fig 4-5c Teeth isolated with a rubber dam. The lingual surfaces are pumiced and the interproximal surfaces are stripped.

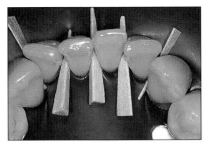

Fig 4-5d Wedges placed to limit the extent of resin interproximally. The lingual surfaces are etched and rinsed, and a fourth-generation (multiple bottle) or fifth-generation (single bottle) enamel-dentin bonding system is applied to the etched lingual surfaces.

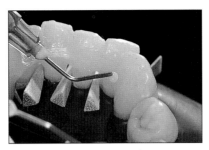

Fig 4-5e Flowable particulate composite resin being applied to the etched lingual surfaces.

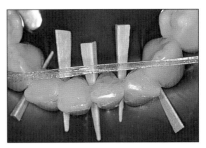

Fig 4-5f Premeasured and cut Splint-It unidirectional FRC material positioned to be tacked into the lingual particulate composite resin.

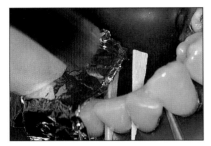

Fig 4-5g The FRC splint material being foil-protected to prevent polymerization of the nonembedded section during light curing of an embedded segment. This technique allows the clinician adequate working time to properly place and embed the FRC along the arch in a sequential manner for maximum adaptation.

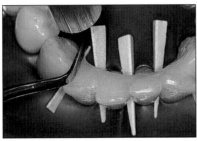

Fig 4-5h A plastic instrument being used to embed the FRC and hold the terminal segment while it is being light polymerized. The FRC must be completely embedded in the particulate composite to protect the glass fibers from oral exposure.

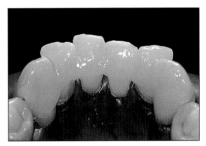

Fig 4-5i Lingual view of the extracoronal FRC splinted mandibular anterior arch. The particulate composite is contoured for comfort if necessary.

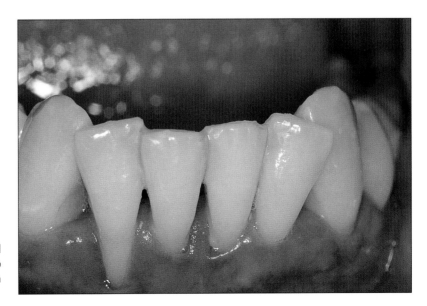

Fig 4-5j Facial view of the extracoronal FRC splinted teeth. When compared to Fig 4–5a, there is no visual indication that the teeth have been splinted.

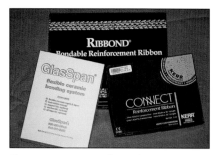

Fig 4-6 Commercially available non–pre-impregnated FRC materials.

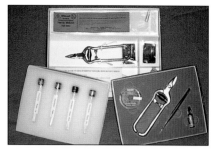

Fig 4-7 Commercially available non–pre-impregnated FRC materials showing contents of boxes. *(Left to right)* GlasSpan, Ribbond, Connect.

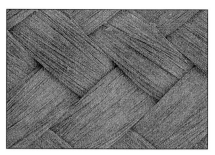

Fig 4-8 Scanning electron micrograph of GlasSpan Rope. (Original magnification × 100.)

Non–pre-impregnated FRC Splinting Technique

Non–pre-impregnated materials include plasma-treated, woven, polyethylene ribbons (Ribbond Reinforcement Ribbon, Ribbond; Connect, Kerr) and flexible white continuous filament glass ceramic fiber that has been etched and silanated (GlasSpan, GlasSpan) (Figs 4-6 and 4-7).

Plasma treatment of the polyethylene ribbon permits a chemical union to take place between the resin and the polyethylene fibers. Etching and silanation of the glass allow for both a mechanical and a chemical union of the fibers. The Ribbond Reinforcement Ribbon is available in a 1.0-mm width for orthodontic stabilization and 2.0-, 3.0-, and 4.0-mm widths for tooth stabilization and tooth replacement. Connect is available in 2.0- and 3.0-mm widths. GlasSpan is available in 1.0-, 1.5-, and 2.0-mm-wide braided ropes (Fig 4-8) and a 2.0-mm-wide woven tape.

Fabrication of a periodontal splint with non–pre-impregnated FRC material is shown in Fig 4-9. The materials used for this chairside procedure are the same as for the pre-impregnated FRC splinting technique with the exception of the type of FRC material that is used.

Fig 4-9 *Fabrication of a periodontal splint with non–pre-impregnated FRC material. (Case courtesy of Dr H.E. Strassler.)*

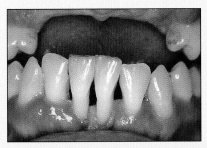

Fig 4-9a Preoperative facial view of mandibular anterior teeth requiring stabilization.

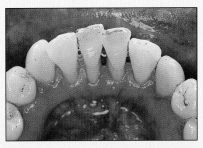

Fig 4-9b Preoperative lingual view of mandibular anterior teeth.

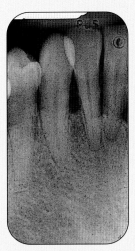
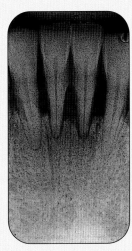
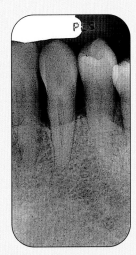

Fig 4-9c Radiographic presentation of the mandibular anterior teeth showing over 70% bone loss.

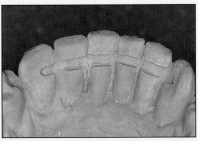

Fig 4-9d Example of channel preparation for ribbon reinforcement in a study cast. The channel dimensions should be the same width and depth as that of the ribbon being used.

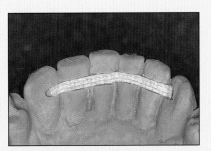

Fig 4-9e Polyethylene ribbon placed into prepared channel. Note that there is no excess length, and the ribbon fills the entire width of the channel.

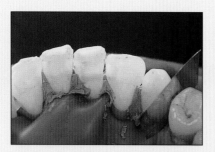

Fig 4-9f A heavy-bodied polyvinyl siloxane impression material being used to block out the gingival embrasures so as to minimize excess composite resin into the embrasures. The purpose of the metal matrix on the distal of the canine is to protect the premolar from being etched. The 2-mm wide by 1-mm deep lingual channel is prepared from canine to canine. The channel is etched and rinsed, and a fourth-generation dentin bonding primer and adhesive is applied. A flowable or hybrid particulate composite is placed into the channel; the resin-impregnated leno-weave polyethylene ribbon is placed into the particulate composite bed; and the splint is visible-light polymerized for 60 seconds over each splinted tooth. If necessary, additional particulate composite is added to completely cover the polyethylene ribbon, and finished to contour.

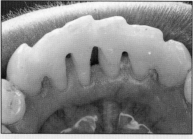

Fig 4-9g Lingual view of completed leno-weave polyethylene ribbon intracoronal splint.

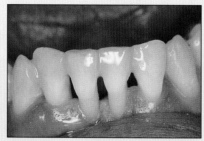

Fig 4-9h Facial view of completed splint giving a very esthetic and imperceptible result. (Compare to Fig 4-9a.)

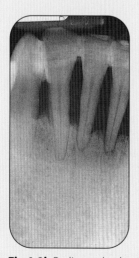
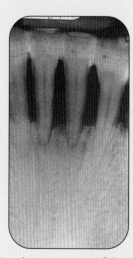
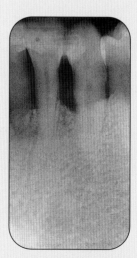

Fig 4-9i Radiographs showing the appearance of the composite resin–polyethylene intracoronal splint. Compare with the preoperative radiographs (Fig 4-9c) and note the appearance of the channel as a result of the radiopaque particulate composite resin that was used.

Fig 4-10 Chairside FRC prosthesis procedure.

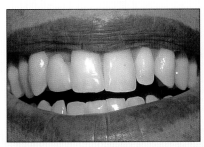
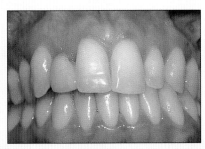
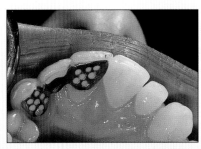

Figs 4-10a and 4-10b Preoperative facial view of a patient with a failing Rochette bridge from the maxillary right central incisor to the canine. Patient was also unhappy about the shape of the left lateral incisor and the canines.

Fig 4-10c Lingual view of failing Rochette bridge from the maxillary right central incisor to the canine.

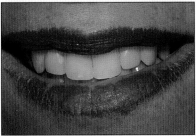
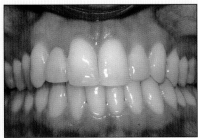
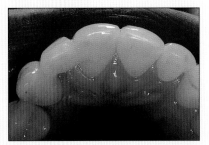

Figs 4-10d and 4-10e Facial views of completed chairside denture tooth pontic FPD. The left lateral incisor has been reshaped with particulate composite resin, and both canines have been recontoured using enamelplasty.

Fig 4-10f Lingual view of chairside denture tooth pontic FPD.

Chairside Conservative Tooth Replacement

Chairside tooth replacement is an excellent application for FRC technology. Previous attempts at chairside tooth replacement involved the use of pontics derived from extracted teeth,[1,2,12,35,41] acrylic resin denture teeth with or without lingual wire reinforcement,[6,13,22,30,45] and resin composite.[12,17,35–37,39–42] These were attached to abutment teeth with acid-etched bonded particulate composite, acid-etched particulate composite, and either wire designs or plasma-treated, polyethylene fiber ribbon. The abutment teeth used for these approaches were usually not prepared; most often, tooth replacement was only for the anterior region and the procedure was considered a short-term solution.

The chairside FRC prosthesis offers a fast, minimally invasive approach for tooth replacement that combines all of the benefits of the FRC material for an esthetic, functional, and potentially durable result (Fig 4-10). A denture tooth or a natural tooth (in the case of an extraction of a periodontally involved incisor) can be used as the pontic.

Selection criteria for this tooth replacement approach include:

- A patient who desires an immediate, minimally invasive approach
- A patient who requires an extraction in an esthetic area and desires an immediate replacement
- Abutment teeth with a questionable long-term prognosis
- Anterior disarticulation during mandibular protrusive movements
- A nonbruxing patient
- Cost considerations

Materials required for the chairside FRC prosthesis procedure are as follows:

- Diagnostic casts
- Denture or natural tooth
- Intraoral putty occlusal-incisal pontic index
- Phosphoric acid gel etchant
- Fourth-generation (multiple bottle) or fifth-generation (single bottle) enamel-dentin bonding system
- Visible light–curing flowable particulate composite
- Unidirectional pre-impregnated FRC
- Finishing and polishing burs and points

Chairside Fixed Partial Denture

Figures 4-11 and 4-12 demonstrate chairside posterior and anterior FRC fixed partial denture (FPD) procedures.

Initial Visit

During the initial visit, a shade is selected for the denture tooth, and an alginate impression of the arch in which the FPD will be placed is taken to create a diagnostic cast. This diagnostic cast is used for selecting and modifying the denture tooth pontic.

Denture Tooth Modification

A denture tooth of appropriate shade that best fits the shape of the edentulous space and that matches the anatomic shape of the adjacent teeth is selected. It is modified so as to lightly contact the proximal surfaces of the abutment teeth and to conform to the ridge of the edentulous space. The denture tooth is then tacked to the cast in an optimal position and a line is inscribed on its occlusal/lingual surface to indicate where the slots are to be placed in the abutment teeth at the time of insertion (Figs 4-11c to 4-11e and 4-12b to 4-12c). The adjusted denture tooth is modified as follows (1) Proximal Class III preparations are placed on the

mesial and distal facial surfaces. These will be used to tack the denture tooth interproximally to the abutment teeth when first positioned in the mouth. (2) An occlusal/lingual groove, at least 2 mm wide and 2 mm deep, is prepared, with the base undercut following the occlusal/lingual line drawn earlier. This groove will receive the FRC (Figs 4-11f and 4-12d).

Alternative Technique Using Extracted Tooth

If the natural tooth is unsalvagable and must be extracted, it can be used as the pontic. The length of the tooth is determined by measuring from the extraction site to the incisal edge of the adjacent teeth; the root is then cut from the tooth crown at this determined length. The root canal opening at the apical end is restored by preparing the root canal with a 330 bur to a depth of 1.5 mm. The preparation is restored with particulate composite using an adhesive technique. The technique for placing the natural tooth crown is similar to that for a denture tooth.

Fabrication of an Intraoral, Occlusal-Incisal Pontic Index

The denture tooth is positioned on the diagnostic cast and a positioning index is fabricated to aid in the accurate alignment of the denture tooth pontic in the mouth. Fabricated from vinyl siloxane putty, the positioning index encompasses the occlusal-incisal portion of the pontic and the adjacent abutment teeth and fills the occlusal/lingual groove for the FRC. The gingival extension should not block facial access to the Class III proximal retentive forms of the pontic (Figs 4-11g to 4-11h and 4-12h).

Chairside Insertion Technique

The abutment teeth are anesthetized; the denture tooth is tried in to verify fit, shade, and contour; and a rubber dam is placed. Grooves are prepared in the abutment teeth to align with the groove in the denture tooth (Figs 4-11k and

Fig 4-11 Chairside posterior FPD procedures using FRC materials.

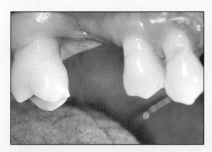

Fig 4-11a Buccal view of edentulous span. Teeth were periodontally compromised and had a questionable long-term prognosis.

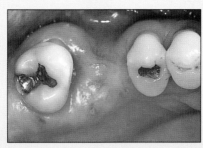

Fig 4-11b Occlusal view of edentulous span.

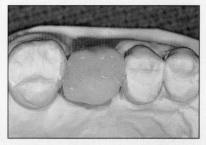

Fig 4-11c Denture tooth pontic luted in place on maxillary cast.

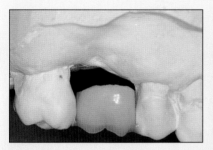

Fig 4-11d Discrepancy between cervical surface of denture tooth and ridge. To obtain a modified ridge lap design, composite resin was built up on the tissue side of the denture tooth.

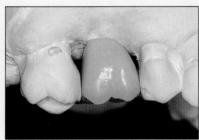

Fig 4-11e Denture tooth pontic with cervical surface modified to fit ridge.

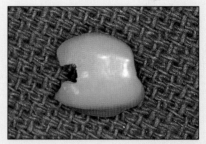

Fig 4-11f Proximal view of the modified denture tooth pontic with occlusal FRC slot in place.

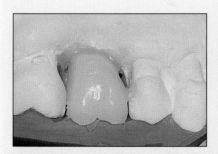

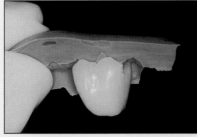

Figs 4-11g and 4-11h Intraoral occlusal pontic positioning index. Note that this design wraps to the lingual and allows unobstructed access to the pontic and abutment teeth from the facial. Putty is locked into the groove so the pontic is stabilized during intraoral insertion.

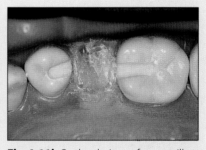

Fig 4-11i Occlusal view of a cast illustrating the slot design in the abutment teeth for this chairside FPD. The dimensions are at least 2 mm wide by 2 mm deep to allow room for 3 to 4 layers of FRC material and an occlusal layer of particulate composite resin.

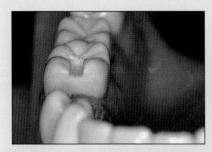

Fig 4-11j Proximal view of occlusal slot. Note that there is no proximal step in this preparation.

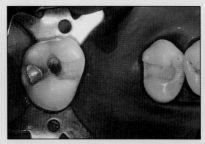

Fig 4-11k Abutment teeth isolated with prepared occlusal slots. The existing amalgam teeth were incorporated into the slot design.

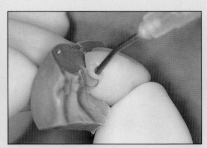

Fig 4-11l Modified denture tooth held in place by the intraoral positioning index. The flowable particulate composite resin is applied to the proximal Class III retentive preparations.

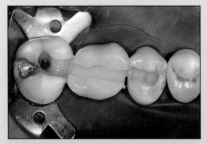

Fig 4-11m Pontic tacked to the abutment teeth with flowable particulate composite, which was placed into the Class III retentive preparations in the pontic and onto the proximal surfaces of the abutment teeth.

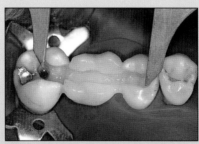

Fig 4-11n Slot length measured for the FRC material.

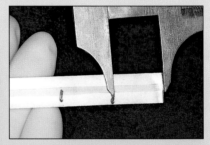

Fig 4-11o Slot length being transferred to the pre-impregnated FRC material, Splint-It, which is encased in its protective paper.

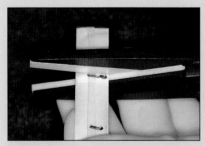

Fig 4-11p The FRC strip being cut using special ceramic scissors, which allow for a clean cut of the glass fibers.

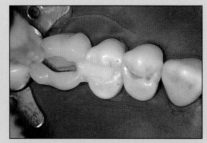

Fig 4-11q High-viscosity flowable particulate composite resin placed into and along the length of the etched and primed occlusal slot.

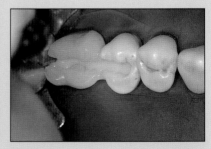

Fig 4-11r High-viscosity particulate composite resin bed in the occlusal slot ready for FRC placement. The particulate composite material is not polymerized prior to FRC placement.

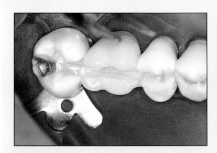

Fig 4-11s Three strips of FRC placed into the composite resin bed within the occlusal slot. Additional particulate composite resin will be added to cover the FRC completely.

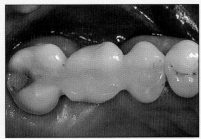

Fig 4-11t Occlusal view of the finished chairside FRC FPD.

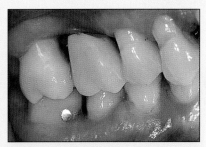

Fig 4-11u Buccal view of the finished chairside FRC FPD.

4-12g); these are to be at least 2 mm wide and 2 mm deep so as to duplicate the groove in the pontic (Figs 4-11i to 4-11j and 4-12f). The occlusal/lingual groove in the denture tooth pontic is sandblasted with 50 μm aluminum oxide. The occlusal/lingual grooves and the interproximal areas of the abutment teeth adjacent to the edentulous space are etched and treated with a dentin bonding agent. The denture tooth is placed in the putty index and positioned in the mouth (Figs 4-11l and 4-12h). A flowable composite is placed and light cured into the Class III interproximal preparations and onto the proximal surfaces of the abutment teeth. This will tack the pontic in place and allow for the removal of the putty index without dislodging or moving the denture tooth

(Figs 4-11m and 4-12i). A small amount of high-viscosity flowable particulate composite resin is syringed into the occlusal/lingual grooves, and the proper length of FRC is added into the particulate composite–based groove (Figs 4-11q and 4-11r). Three or more pieces of FRC should be placed and condensed into the groove, below the occlusal/lingual surface of the abutment teeth or pontic, and then light cured (Fig 4-11s). A less viscous flowable particulate composite resin is used to completely fill the remaining portion of the groove and light cured (Figs 4-11t and 4-12k to 4-12l). The rubber dam is removed and occlusal adjustments are made using a high-speed handpiece with a composite finishing bur.

Fig 4-12 *Chairside anterior FPD procedures using FRC materials.*

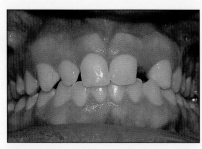

Fig 4-12a Patient presenting with missing left lateral incisor and peg-shaped right lateral incisor.

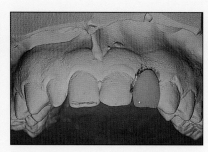

Fig 4-12b Facial view of modified denture tooth on maxillary cast.

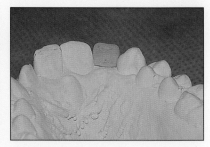

Fig 4-12c Lingual view of modified denture tooth on maxillary cast.

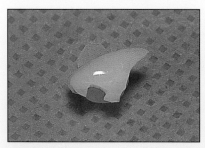

Fig 4-12d Proximal view of the lingual FRC slot prepared on the modified denture tooth.

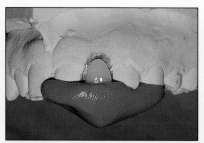

Fig 4-12e Intraoral incisal pontic positioning index with denture tooth on the maxillary cast. Note that the index allows access to the interproximal surfaces of the denture tooth and abutments.

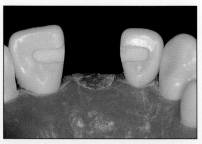

Fig 4-12f Cast with lingual slot preparations. Slots must be at least 2 mm wide, 2 mm long, and 2 mm deep to receive at least 3 to 4 strips of FRC material.

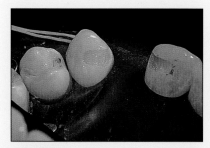

Fig 4-12g Rubber dam isolation with the lingual slots prepared on the central incisor and the canine.

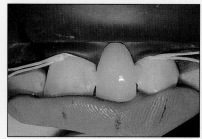

Fig 4-12h Intraoral incisal pontic positioning index in place, aligning the denture tooth pontic in the correct position. Particulate composite resin has been added interproximally to tack the pontic prior to removal of the index. This will hold the pontic for the placement of the FRC.

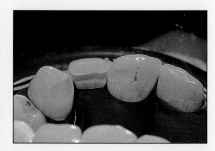

Fig 4-12i Lingual view of the tacked pontic, ready for FRC placement. Note the alignment of the pontic groove with the slots on the canine and the central incisor.

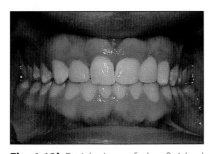

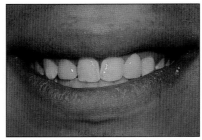

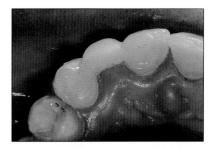

Fig 4-12j Facial view of the finished chairside FRC FPD and recontoured peg-shaped right lateral incisor. Note the excellent ridge adaptation of the pontic.

Fig 4-12k Facial view with smile. Note the natural appearance of the final result.

Fig 4-12l Lingual view of the completed chairside FRC fixed prosthesis. The lingual contour has not been altered by the FRC placement.

Endodontic FRC Posts

FRC posts are a recent addition to the systems traditionally used to retain a core in severely broken down, endodontically treated teeth: custom-made metal or cast posts and cores and prefabricated metal and zirconium posts. The FRC posts offer greater flexure and fatigue strength, a modulus of elasticity close to that of dentin, the ability to form a single bonded complex within the root canal for a unified root-post complex, and improved esthetics when used with all-ceramic or FRC crowns as compared to custom-made cast or metal-prefabricated posts.[11,15,16,19,27,31,38,45] The properties of this post design have the potential to reinforce a compromised root and to distribute stress more uniformly on loading to prevent root fracture; moreover, the FRC post will yield prior to catastrophic root failure better than will custom-made cast metal or prefabricated metal post systems.[18,24,25,47]

Two categories of FRC posts are available: chairside-fabricated and prefabricated. Chairside-fabricated posts are custom designs that use polyethylene non–pre-impregnated woven fibers (Ribbond, Connect) or glass fibers (GlasSpan) to reinforce the root and hold a composite core.[11,18] Prefabricated posts (Fig 4-13) are constructed of two kinds of fiber: carbon fibers embedded in an epoxy matrix (C-Post, U-M C-Post, and Aestheti-Post) (Figs 4-14 to 4-16)[4,5,7–9,24] and S-type glass fibers embedded in a filled resin matrix (FibreKor Post) (Fig 4-17).[27]

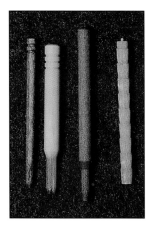

Fig 4-13 The 4 designs of preformed FRC posts *(left to right)*: U-M C-Post, Aestheti-Post, C-Post, FibreKor Post.

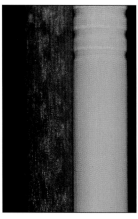

Fig 4-14 Carbon fiber post shafts: C-Post *(left)* and Aestheti-Post *(right)*. The exterior of the Aestheti-Post is coated with a tooth-colored mineral sheath to mask the dark carbon color. (Original magnification × 10.)

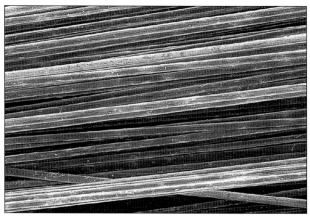

Fig 4-15 Scanning electron micrograph of carbon fibers from a C-Post. The epoxy matrix has been removed. These fibers are 8 μm in diameter and constitute 64% of the post by weight. (Original magnification × 500.)

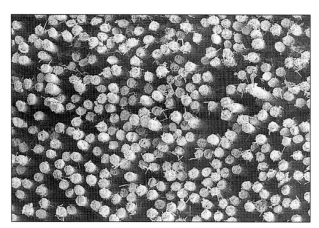

Fig 4-16 Scanning electron micrograph of cross section of carbon fibers from a C-Post. The epoxy has been removed. (Original magnification × 500.)

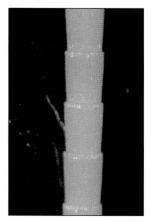

Fig 4-17 FibreKor Post. The surface appears to be less irregular compared to the carbon fiber posts and has a resin coating. The composition of the post by weight percent is 42% glass fiber, 29% filler, and 29% resin. (Original magnification × 10.)

Fig 4-18 *Chairside prefabricated and fabricated FRC post procedure.*

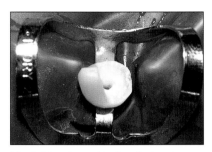

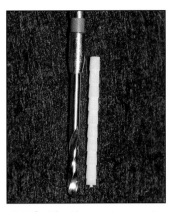

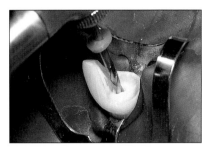

Fig 4-18a Central incisor, isolated to receive a glass fiber FibreKor Post in preparation for a pressed ceramic crown.

Fig 4-18b FibreKor post space is prepared in one step using a post drill sized for the selected post width.

Fig 4-18c Preparation of post space to the selected depth.

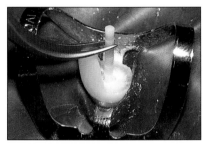

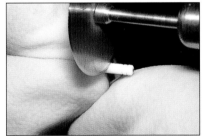

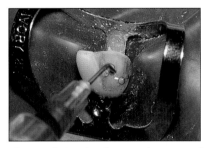

Fig 4-18d FibreKor Post try-in. It should seat passively and should not bind against the canal walls.

Fig 4-18e The post is cut, using either a diamond wheel, diamond bur, or carbide bur, to a height that will allow it to completely support the particulate composite resin core. FRC posts should not be cut with scissors or pliers, which would damage the integrity of the resin or epoxy matrix holding the fibers together.

Fig 4-18f Canal and internal aspects of the tooth being etched with phosphoric acid.

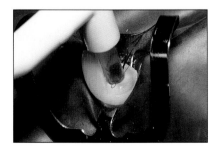

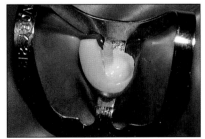

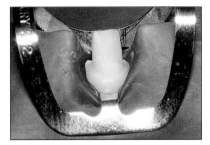

Fig 4-18g A dual-cure or chemical-cure fourth-generation enamel-dentin bond system applied to the canal and chamber dentin.

Fig 4-18h The post cemented using a dual-cure particulate composite resin luting. The canal should be lined and the apical third of the post coated with the particulate composite resin cement.

Fig 4-18i The particulate composite resin core with completed tooth preparation (facial view). The shoulder is located at least 1 to 2 mm below the gingival margin of the particulate composite core, on sound tooth structure, to create a ferule effect.

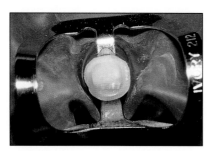

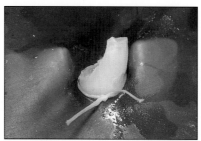

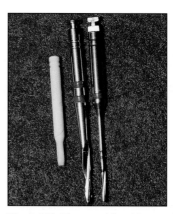

Fig 4-18j FibreKor Post and composite resin core with completed tooth preparation (incisal view). The end of the post can be seen through the lingual incisal of the core.

Fig 4-18k Central incisor, isolated to receive a carbon fiber Aestheti-Post in preparation for a pressed ceramic crown.

Fig 4-18l The canal for this post is prepared in two steps. A preshaping drill *(far right)* is used to prepare the post space to its final depth and to guide the final canal preparation. A finishing drill *(middle)* is used to shape the canal so as to accept the carbon fiber post and to create a 30-mm space for resin cement.

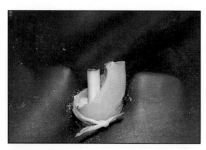

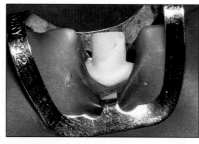

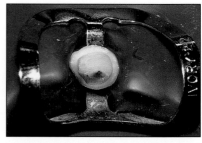

Fig 4-18m Aestheti-Post seated after post space preparation and height adjustment. Note that the height is enough to allow complete extension of the post to provide support for the particulate composite core.

Fig 4-18n Completed Aestheti-Post and particulate composite resin core (facial view).

Fig 4-18o Completed Aestheti-Post and particulate composite resin core with tooth prepared to receive a pressed ceramic crown (incisal view). Note the end of the carbon fiber post on the lingual incisal portion of the core.

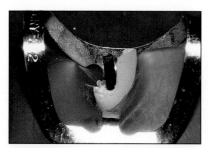

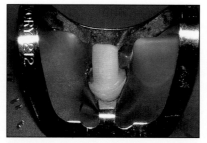

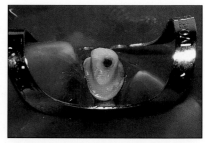

Fig 4-18p A carbon fiber C-Post cemented into a tooth in preparation for a particulate composite resin core (facial view). The same steps followed for the Aestheti-Post placement, above, apply to the C-Post.

Fig 4-18q Finished C-Post and particulate composite resin with completed tooth preparation to receive a pressed ceramic crown (facial view). Depending on the buccolingual width of the composite core, this type of FRC post may result in a core with lower value because of its color.

Fig 4-18r Finished C-Post and particulate composite resin core with completed tooth preparation (incisal view). Note that the C-Post is visible at the lingual incisal edge of the core.

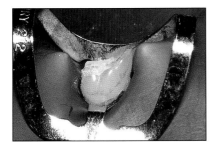

Fig 4-18s Isolation of a central incisor to receive a chairside fabricated FRC post. There is no post space step in this procedure. The canal is used as it was shaped during the filing of the canal prior to obturation.

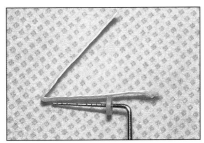

Fig 4-18t The non–pre-impregnated, polyethylene woven ribbon (Ribbond) cut to a length that will allow a "V"-shape for canal insertion and enough height to support the core. A periodontal probe or endodontic explorer or plugger can be used as the placement instrument. The rubber stopper indicates the canal length.

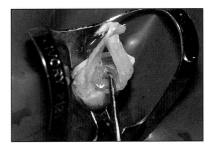

Fig 4-18u The resin-saturated length of polyethylene woven ribbon being placed into the canal, which has previously been etched, primed, filled with adhesive, and lined with a dual-cure particulate composite resin luting cement. Additional lengths of ribbon are placed into the canal until no more can be added.

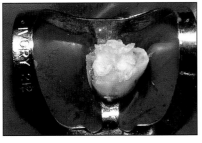

Fig 4-18v The canal maximally obturated with the resin-saturated polyethylene ribbon. The "ears" that are left exposed in the chamber will support the composite core material.

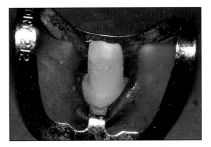

Fig 4-18w Finished chairside fabricated FRC post and particulate composite resin core prepared to receive a pressed ceramic crown (facial view).

FRC Post Selection and Placement Technique

The introduction of the FRC posts has been too recent to allow sufficient data to be gathered to document their successes and failures in certain clinical situations and to permit more than a conservative approach to their use at the present time. The longest reported study involving C-Posts on single anterior and posterior crowns concluded that, over the 3-year observation period, the system "seems to be a promising alternative to conventional cast metallic posts."[9]

With this in mind, the FRC post can be considered for teeth that can have a margin placed below the composite core on sound tooth structure to allow for a ferule effect, and for those teeth with large, flared canals where the composite luting resin–FRC combination can create a bonded, reinforced root. The FRC post potentially offers the clinician the possibility of strengthening the root through adhesive technology, and if failure does occur, it most likely will be at the post-core interface, and not within the tooth or root.[24]

Materials required for the chairside prefabricated/fabricated FRC post procedure, illustrated in Fig 4-18, are as follows:

- Rubber dam, retraction clamps (eg, Ivory 212)
- FRC prefabricated post kit (C-Post, U-M C-Post, Aestheti-Post, FibreKor Post) or polyethylene woven ribbon (Ribbond, Connect)
- Peeso reemers, endodontic pluggers, alcohol lamp/bunsen burner, to remove gutta-purcha from canal(s)
- Fourth-generation dual-cure or chemical-cure dentin bonding system
- Dual-cure composite luting resin
- Particulate composite resin core paste

Step-by-Step Prefabricated FRC Post and Core Procedure

1. Using a rubber dam and a gingival retraction clamp (eg, Ivory 212) or floss ligation, isolate the tooth.
2. Using either heat or a Peeso reemer, remove gutta-percha from within the canal to 4 to 5 mm of apex.
3. Using proper drills, select the size of prefabricated posts to fit within the canal and select proper size preparation drills and post hole preparation.
4. Using either a diamond disk or a diamond bur, cut the selected, fitted post to the correct height.
5. Etch and rinse the root canal, chamber, and remaining tooth structure, and apply a fourth-generation chemical-cure dentin bond primer and adhesive.
6. Coat the FRC post with primer and place a dual-cure or chemical-cure particulate composite resin luting cement into the root canal and on the apical third of the post and insert the post into the canal.
7. Add particulate composite resin core material to the remaining chamber and crown and the core prepared for a crown.

Step-by-Step Fabricated FRC Post and Core Procedure

1. Perform steps 1 and 2, above, for the prefabricated FRC post and core procedure.
2. Do not enlarge or shape the existing canal space, but cut strips of polyethylene woven ribbon in excess of twice the post space.
3. Etch, rinse, and apply a fourth-generation chemical-cure dentin bonding system to the canal space, pulp chamber, and remaining tooth structure.
4. Apply dual-cure or chemical-cure particulate composite resin luting cement into the canal.
5. Saturate the polyethylene woven ribbon with resin, form it into a "V" shape, and place it into the canal, leaving the excess as an "ear" out into the chamber/remaining tooth structure. Place as many pieces of polyethylene woven ribbon as will fit into the canal.
6. Apply particulate composite resin core material to the polyethylene woven ribbon coronal extensions to create a core and prepare a crown preparation of the core-tooth complex.

Acknowledgment

Dr H.E. Strassler contributed the series of slides and text that appear on pages 57–58.

References

1. Antonoson DE. Immediate temporary bridge using an extracted tooth. Dent Surv 1980:22;208–211.
2. Bounocore MG. The uses of adhesives in dentistry. Springfield IL: Charles C Thomas, 1975:334.
3. Ciancio SG, Nisengard RJ. Resins in periodontal splinting. Dent Clin North Am 1975;19(2):235–242.
4. Composiposte. Technical document: Meylan Cedex, France RTD; 1994.
5. Dallari A, Rovatti L. Six years of in vitro/in vivo experience with Composipost. Compend Contin Educ Dent 1996;17(S20):S58.

6. Davila JM, Gwinnett AV. Clinical and microscopic evaluation of a bridge using the acid-etch technique (ASDC). J Dent Child 1978;45:52–54.

7. Duret B, Reynaud M, Duret F. New concept of coronoradicular reconstruction: The Composiposte (part 1). Chir Dent France 1990;60(540):131–141.

8. Duret B, Duret G, Reynaud M. Long life physical property preservation and postendodontic rehabilitation with the Composipost. Compend Contin Educ Dent 1996;17(S20): S50–S56.

9. Fredriksson M, Astback J, Pamenius M, Arvidson K. A retrospective study of 236 patients with teeth restored by carbon fiber-reinforced epoxy resin posts. J Prosthet Dent 1998;80(2):151–157.

10. Greenfield DS, Nathanson D. Periodontal splinting with wire and composite resin. A revised approach. J Periodontol 1980;51(8):465–468.

11. Hornbrook D, Hastings RJ. Use of bondable reinforcement fiber for post and core build-up in an endodontically treated tooth: Maximizing strength and aesthetics. Pract Periodontics Aesthet Dent 1995;7(5):33–42.

12. Ibsen RL. Fixed prosthetics with a natural crown pontic using adhesive composite. J South Calif Dent Assoc 1973;41:100–103.

13. Ibsen RL, Neville K. Adhesive restorative dentistry. Philadelphia: WB Saunders, 1974:139.

14. Inguez I, Strassler HE. Polyethylene ribbon and fixed orthodontic retention and porcelain veneers: Solving an esthetic dilemma. J Esthet Dent 1998;10:52–59.

15. Isador F, Brondum K. Intermittent loading of teeth with tapered, individual cast or prefabricated parallel-sided posts. Int J Prosthodont 1992;5:257–261.

16. Isador F, Odman P, Brondum K. Intermittent loading of teeth restored using prefabricated carbon fiber posts. Int J Prosthodont 1996;9:131–136.

17. Jensen ME, Meiers JC. Resin-Bonded Retainers in Clinical Dentistry, vol 4. Philadelphia: Harper and Row, 1984:4–5.

18. Karna JC. A fiber composite laminate endodontic post and core. Am J Dent 1996;9(5):230–232.

19. King PA, Setchell KJ. An in vitro evaluation of a prototype CFRC prefabricated post developed for the restoration of pulpless teeth. J Oral Rehabil 1990; 17:599–609.

20. Klassman B, Zucker HW. Combination wire-composite intracoronal splinting rationale and technique. J Periodontol 1976;47(8):481–486.

21. Liatukas EL. An amalgam and composite resin splint for posterior teeth. J Prosthet Dent 1973;30(2):173–175.

22. Littman H, Regan D, Rakow B. Provisional temporization with acid-etch resin technique. Clin Prev Dent 1980;2: 14–17.

23. Lloyd RS, Baer PN. Permanent fixed amalgam splints. J Periodont 1959;30:163.

24. Martinez-Insua A, Da Silva L, Rilo B, Santana U. Comparison of fracture resistance of pulpless teeth restored with a cast post-and-core or carbon-fiber post with a composite core. J Prosthet Dent 1998;80:527–532.

25. Mentink AG, Meenwisser R, Kayser AF, Mulder J. Survival rate and failure characteristics of the all metal post and core restoration. J Oral Rehabil 1993;20:455–461.

26. Miller TE. A new material for periodontal splinting and orthodontic retention. Compend Cont Educ Dent 1993;14:800–812.

27. Nash RW. The use of posts for endodontically treated teeth. Compend Contin Educ Dent 1998;19(10): 1054–1062.

28. Obin JN, Arvins AN. The use of self-curing resin splints for temporary stabilization of mobile teeth due to periodontal involvement. J Am Dent Assoc 1951;42:320.

29. Oikarinen K. Tooth splinting: A review of the literature and consideration of the versatility of a wire-composite splint. Endod Dent Traumatol 1990;6(6):237–250.

30. Portnoy L. Constructing a composite pontic in a single visit. Dent Surv 1973;49(8):20–23.

31. Purton DG, Love RM. Rigidity and retention of carbon fiber versus stainless steel root canal posts. Int Endod J 1996;29:262–265.

32. Saravanamuttu R. Post-orthodontic splinting of periodontally involved teeth. Br J Orthod 1990;17(1): 29–32.

33. Schmid MO, Lutz F, Imfeld T. A new reinforced intracoronal composite resin splint. Clinical results after 1 year. J Periodontol 1979;50(9):441–444.

34. Schwarz MS, Sochat P. The interim intracoronal wire and acrylic splint. J South Calif Dent Assoc 1972;40(12): 1067–1069.

35. Simonsen RJ. Clinical Applications of the Acid Etch Technique. Chicago: Quintessence, 1978:71–80.

36. Simonsen RJ. The acid etch technique in fixed prostheses. An update. Quintessence Int 1980;9:33–40

37. Simonsen R, Thompson V, Barrack G. Etched Cast Restorations: Clinical and Laboratory Techniques. Chicago: Quintessence, 1983.

38. Sorenson JA, Engelmen MJ. Effect of post adaptation on fracture resistance of endodontically treated teeth. J Prosthet Dent 1990;64:419–424.

39. Stolpa JB. An adhesive technique for small anterior fixed partial dentures. J Prosthet Dent 1975;34:513–515.

40. Strassler HE, Gerhardt DE. Management of restorative emergencies. Dent Clin North Am 1993;37:353–366.

41. Strassler HE, LoPresti J, Scherer W, Rudo D. Clinical evaluation of a woven polyethylene ribbon used for splinting. Esthet Dent Update 1995;6:80–84.

42. Strassler HE. Planing with diagnostic casts for success with direct composite bonding. J Esthet Dent 1995;7(1):32–40.

43. Strassler HE, Serio FG. Stabilization of the natural dentition in periodontal cases using adhesive restorative materials. Perio Insights 1997;4:4–10.

44. Sweeney EJ, Moore DL, Dooner JJ. Retentive strength of acid-etched anterior fixed partial dentures: An in vitro comparison of attachment techniques. J Am Dent Assoc 1980;100:198–201.

45. Torbjorner A, Karlsson S, Syverud M, Hensten-Pettersen A. Carbon fiber reinforced root canal posts. Mechanical and cytotoxic properties. Eur J Oral Sci 1996;104:605–611.

46. Vitsentzos SI, Koidis PT. Facial approach to stabilization of mobile maxillary anterior teeth with steep overlap and occlusal trauma. J Prosthet Dent 1997;77:550–552.

47. Yaman P, Thorsteinsson T. Effects of core materials on stress distribution of posts. J Prosthet Dent 1992;68:416–420.

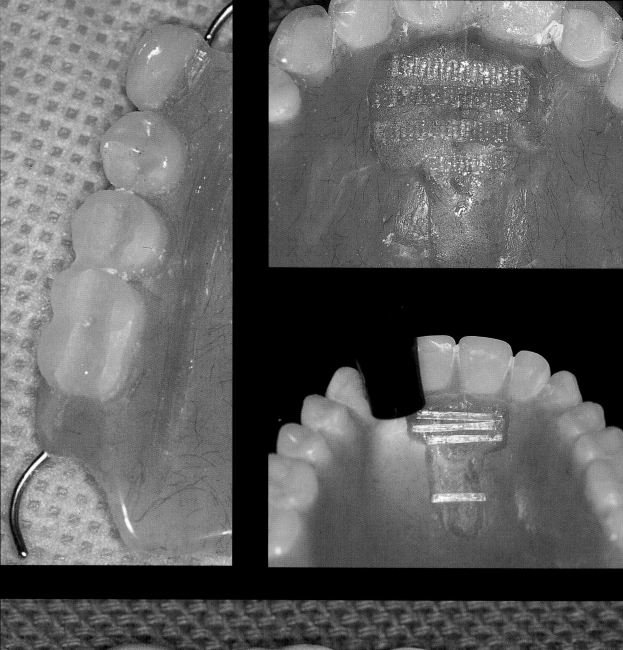
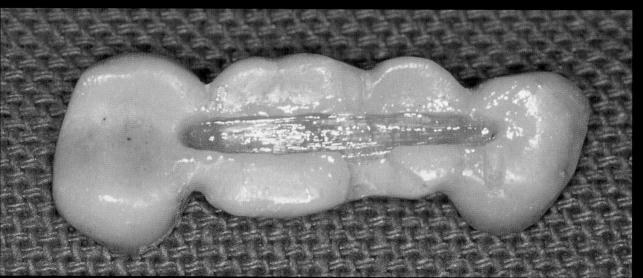

Repair of Acrylic Resin Prostheses

■ For several decades, acrylic resins have been used to fabricate various types of removable prostheses and provisional fixed partial dentures (FPDs). These resins are esthetic and easy to manipulate, and they offer satisfactory mechanical properties; however, fractures resulting from impact and flexural fatigue do occur. Depending on their timing and circumstances, these fractures are inconvenient both for patient and practitioner and potentially disastrous.

Repairs to these prostheses are generally made by applying "band-aid" patches of resin to the site of the fracture. Laboratory studies have documented that these repairs are even weaker than the original prostheses,[1,5,6] and clinical experience has shown that the repaired prosthesis often refractures in the same place within a short period of time.

Wires and metal meshworks have been incorporated into these repairs for the purpose of providing additional reinforcement. However, the parent resin does not bond to these metal alloys, and the nonresin reinforcement merely holds the two pieces of the prosthesis together when it ultimately fractures again.

Until the development of glass fiber–reinforced composites, a predictable, convenient, and esthetic technique for repairing resin prostheses has not been available. Its superior flexure strength, combined with the capacity of its resinous matrix both to uniformly wet the fibers and to chemically bond to the parent resin, makes glass fiber–reinforced composite an ideal material for long-term resin repairs.[2,4]

Both unidirectional and woven light-polymerized FRC strips can be used effectively for chairside repairs of fractured acrylic resin prostheses. As noted in chapter 3, FibreKor (Jeneric/Pentron) and Vectris (Ivoclar/Williams) are unidirectional materials available for laboratory use. Splint-It (Jeneric/Pentron), another chairside material, is available either as a unidirectional or a woven fiber. All of these materials have significantly greater flexural properties than unreinforced resin.[3] As explained earlier, woven FRC has a shorter memory than unidirectional FRC, which makes it easier to handle; however, unidirectional FRC has superior flexural properties and will likely provide a stronger repair.

Indications and Procedures for Chairside Repairs with Light-polymerized FRC

Virtually any acrylic resin prosthesis or appliance can be repaired with light-polymerized FRC:

- Complete dentures
- Acrylic bases of partial dentures
- Provisional removable partial dentures
- Provisional FPDs
- Obturators
- Palatal lift appliances
- Orthodontic retainers
- Occlusal splints and night guards

Techniques for repairing partial and total fractures of complete dentures are illustrated in Figs 5-1 and 5-2, respectively. The same set of principles can easily be applied to any of the situations listed above, with positive results. Repair of a provisional FPD is shown in Fig 5-3.

Materials required for chairside repair of acrylic resin prostheses are as follows:

- Low-speed handpiece and acrylic burs
- Visible light–curing flowable composite resin
- Pre-impregnated FRC material (unidirectional or woven)
- Ceramic scissors
- Visible light–curing unit
- Acrylic resin (parent material or other applicable self-polymerizing resin)
- Paintbrush/dappen dishes
- Ruler
- Pressure pot
- Pumice wheel and lathe

If the prosthesis or appliance is completely fractured, the following additional items will be needed:

- Sticky wax
- Cyanoacrylate
- Dental stone

Fig 5-1 Step-by-step procedure for the repair of a partially fractured acrylic resin maxillary denture using light-polymerized FRC.

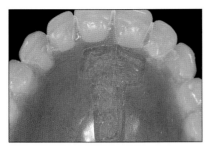

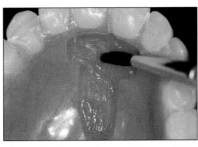

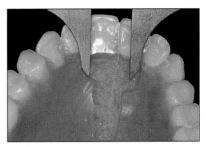

Fig 5-1a If the denture (or other removable resin prosthesis/appliance) is cracked but still in one piece, a T-shaped cavity approximately 1.5 to 2.0 mm deep is created over the crack.

Fig 5-1b The surface of the cavity is prepared by wetting it first with acrylic resin monomer and then with special resin (Jeneric/Pentron). This resin layer is not polymerized, and it creates an adhesive surface that allows for the FRC to be "tacked down."

Fig 5-1c The width of the cavity is measured.

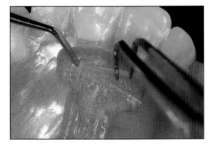

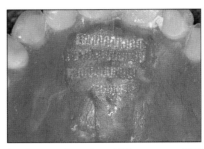

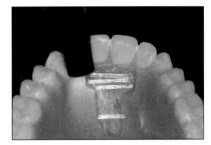

Figs 5-1d and 5-1e Four or more strips of either unidirectional (d) or woven FRC (e) are cut to size and placed horizontally over the fracture.

Fig 5-1f The FRC is light polymerized for 4 minutes.

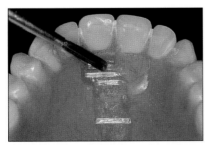

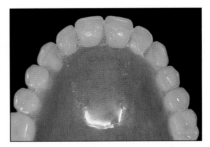

Fig 5-1g The remainder of the cavity is filled with acrylic resin.

Fig 5-1h The prosthesis is placed in a pressure pot at 20 psi with warm water. After 15 minutes, the prosthesis is removed, pumiced, and polished.

Fig 5-2 Step-by-step procedure for the repair of a completely fractured acrylic resin maxillary denture using light-polymerized FRC.

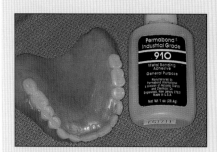

Fig 5-2a The two fractured halves of the prosthesis are rejoined with cyanoacrylate and sticky wax.

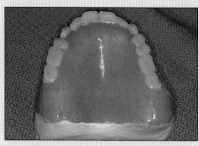

Fig 5-2b A stone cast is poured into the prosthesis after any undercuts are blocked out. This cast will maintain the orientation of the two segments throughout the repair.

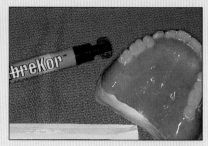

Fig 5-2c The entire area of the fracture is opened with a carbide bur. The surface of the fracture site is then prepared first with acrylic monomer and then with unpolymerized special liquid resin.

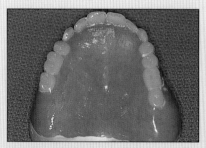

Fig 5-2d Multiple strips of FRC are cut and tacked across the fracture site and then light cured.

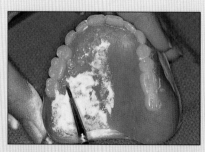

Fig 5-2e The FRC repair is then covered with resin.

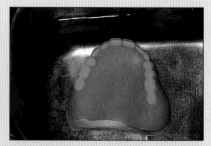

Fig 5-2f The prosthesis is placed in warm water and allowed to polymerize for 15 minutes in a pressure pot at 20 psi.

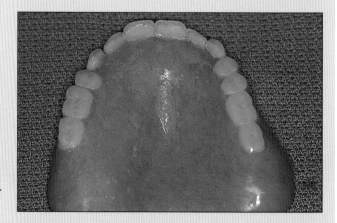

Fig 5-2g After the prosthesis is polished, it is ready for delivery.

Fig 5-3 Step-by-step procedure for the repair of a fractured acrylic resin provisional FPD using light-polymerized FRC.

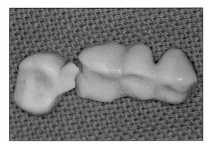

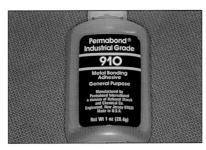

Fig 5-3a Any short- or long-span provisional FPD may be repaired with FRC.

Figs 5-3b and 5-3c The two halves of the provisional FPD are rejoined with cyanoacrylate.

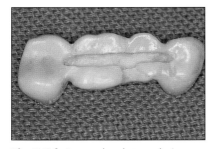

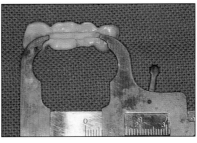

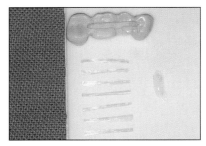

Fig 5-3d An occlusal trough is prepared across the fracture and connecting the abutments. If possible, the trough should be approximately 2 mm deep and 2 mm wide.

Fig 5-3e The length of the trough is measured. The parent resin is then prepared as before with monomer and unpolymerized special liquid resin.

Fig 5-3f Multiple strips of FRC are cut to the proper length.

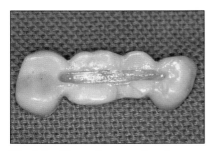

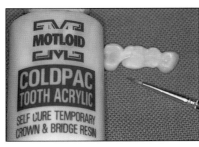

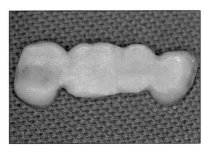

Fig 5-3g The strips are placed across the fracture site and then light cured for 4 minutes.

Fig 5-3h The FRC repair is covered with resin.

Fig 5-3i After it is cured in a pressure pot (desirable, but not required), the prosthesis is polished and is then ready for delivery.

Fig 5-4 *Modification of a transitional partial denture from complete to partial palatal coverage.*

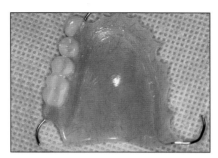

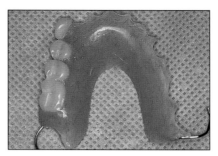

Fig 5-4a Trough created to allow for the placement of FRC. Several strips of FRC are measured, cut, placed, cured, and then covered with resin.

Fig 5-4b The final result after the palate has been opened and the prosthesis polished.

Reinforcement of Provisional Acrylic Resin Prostheses

The technique illustrated in Fig 5-3 for the repair of a provisional FPD can also be used to reinforce a provisional FPD before delivery, which can help to prevent fractures. Reinforcement can be extremely useful with long-span provisional FPDs in patients with destructive parafunctional habits and when only minimal space is available for the acrylic resin.

Figure 5-4 illustrates the procedure for converting a full palatal-coverage transitional partial denture to a horseshoe-shaped removable prosthesis. Placing FRC allows acrylic bases to be reduced to the smallest dimensions possible, which would fracture without reinforcement. The minimal dimensions can be a significant advantage for patients who cannot tolerate the bulk of a traditional transitional partial denture.

The development of pre-impregnated glass fiber–reinforced composites has provided a simple, esthetic, and reliable mechanism for repairing and reinforcing most prostheses fabricated with acrylic resin. The simple and straightforward procedures and materials presented in this chapter can easily be incorporated into office practice for the clinician or trained auxiliary staff.

References

1. Berge M. Bending strength of intact and repaired denture base resin. Acta Odontol Scand 1983;41:187–191.

2. Freilich MA, Karmaker AC, Burstone CJ, Goldberg AJ. Flexure strength and handling characteristics of fiber-reinforced composites used in prosthodontics [abstract 1361]. J Dent Res 1997;76:184.

3. Freilich MA, Karmaker AC, Burstone CJ, Goldberg AJ. Flexure strength of fiber-reinforced composites designed for prosthodontic application [abstract 999]. J Dent Res 1997;76:138.

4. Goldberg AJ, Burstone CJ. The use of continuous fiber reinforcement in dentistry. Dent Mater 1992;8:197–202.

5. Koumjian JH, Nimmo A. Evaluation of fracture resistance of resins used for provisional restorations. J Prosthet Dent 1990;64:654–657.

6. Vallitu PK, Lassial VP, Lappalainen R. Wetting the repair surface with methyl methacrylate affects the transverse strength of repaired heat-polymerized resin. J Prosthet Dent 1994;72:639–643.

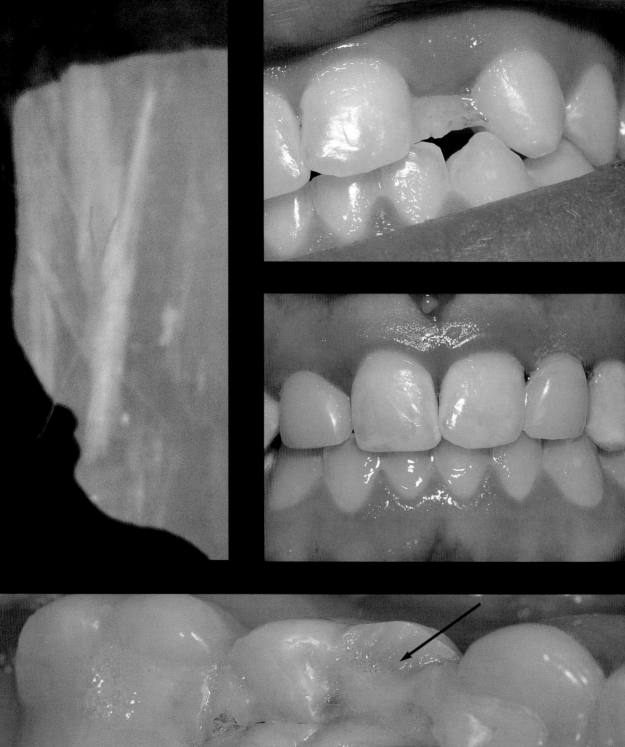
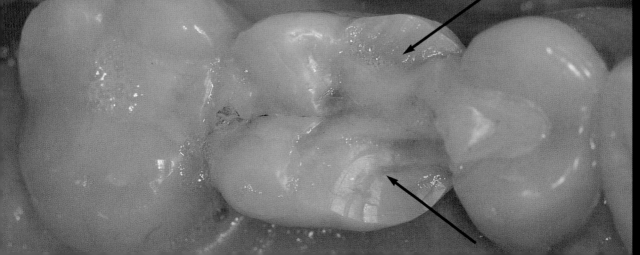

Managing Clinical Problems

■ The problems a clinician may experience with fiber-reinforced composite (FRC) fixed partial dentures (FPDs) can be grouped under the following categories:

- Gray/metal showthrough of metal posts and cores or amalgam cores on abutment teeth
- Loss of surface luster on the particulate composite veneer
- Excessive translucency in pontic areas
- Low concentration of veneer color (chroma), particularly in pontic areas
- Sensitivity after cementation
- Fracture of the particulate composite veneer
- Debonding of the retainer

Gray/Metal Showthrough of Metal Posts and Cores or Amalgam Cores on Abutment Teeth

While enhancing esthetics, the translucency of the FRC framework and veneering particulate composite can make it difficult to mask the underlying metal (Fig 6-1). This problem can be solved in a number of ways. One solution is not to use cast metal posts and cores or amalgam cores on abutment teeth in combination with an FRC fixed prosthesis. Fiber-reinforced composite posts with composite cores (see chapter 4) and zirconium posts with pressed ceramic cores are the materials of choice for endodontic abutment teeth that require a post and

Fig 6-1 *Patient presenting with metal buildup on left central incisor. The lateral incisor was replaced with an FRC FPD. Graying from the existing amalgam that was placed in the chamber is clearly visible. A metal prefabricated post had been cemented into the canal of the central incisor. A decision was made to leave the existing amalgam core and metal prefabricated post.*

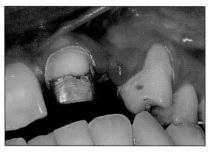 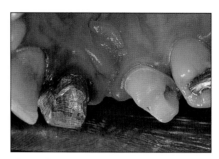 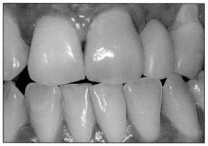

Fig 6-1a Facial view. Teeth were prepared for a full-coverage FRC FPD.

Fig 6-1b Lingual view.

Fig 6-1c Facial view of completed FRC FPD on abutment teeth. Note the graying of the left central incisor from the showthrough of the amalgam core.

core and an FRC retainer. If an existing cast metal post and core or amalgam core is not going to be replaced, a solution is to apply resin opaquers to mask the metal in a shade similar to that chosen for the FRC. In this situation it is also helpful to inform the laboratory that a metal core will be used so that the technician can use opaque shades of veneering particulate composite to decrease the translucency of the retainer.

Loss of Surface Luster of Particulate Composite Veneer

The surface of the veneering particulate composite has shown a tendency to lose its original luster over time. Such loss of luster is apparent in photographs in which the FPD is not bathed

in saliva. Examples of this phenomenon are shown in Figs 6-2 and 6-3. Attempts to restore luster by applying a resin surface glaze or by polishing with points or pastes have not had a lasting effect. Fortunately, the durability of the FRC is not diminished by loss of luster, and there has been no evidence of an increase in visible surface staining associated with this process.

Excessive Translucency in Pontic Areas

Both particulate and FRC materials have the potential to exhibit high translucency. While this characteristic is desirable in retainer areas, it can be an esthetic liability in pontic areas where there is no underlying tooth structure to block light transmission. As illustrated in Fig 6-4,

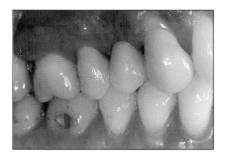

Fig 6-2a Three-unit FRC FPD from the maxillary right second premolar to canine, at cementation. Although saliva-free, the FPD surface has a high polish.

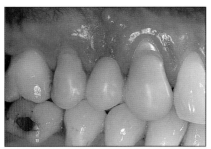

Fig 6-2b FRC FPD at 6-month recall, dry. The surface appears very smooth but without a high polish.

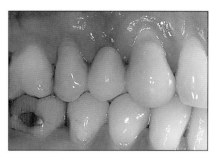

Fig 6-2c FPD at 6-month recall, wetted with saliva. The surface appears to have a high polish, similar to when it was first placed.

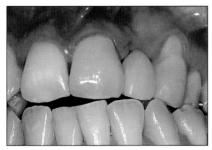

Fig 6-3a Three-unit FRC FPD from the maxillary left central incisor to canine, at cementation. The surface has a high polish.

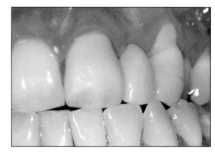

Fig 6-3b FPD at 6-month recall, dry. The surface appears very smooth but without a high polish.

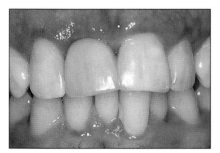

Fig 6-4 Anterior FRC FPD with "grayed" pontic due to excessive translucency.

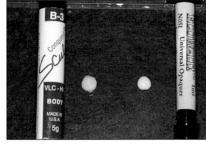

Fig 6-5 Comparison of composite opaque material *(left)* and dentin shade B3.

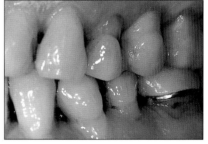

Fig 6-6 Intraoral appearance of an FRC prosthesis that received a thin application of opaque material to reduce translucency of the pontic and reduce grayness. The pontic is the maxillary second premolar.

unimpeded transmission of light through the pontic in the maxillary left central incisor results in a "graying" effect. The application of a thin layer of universal resin opaque material to the FRC framework effectively blocks the unimpeded transmission of light and eliminates the excessive gray appearance of the pontic. The opaque material and its similarity to dentin shade B3 are shown in Fig 6-5. Figure 6-6 shows the final intraoral appearance of an FRC prosthesis that has received an application of opaque material to the pontic framework.

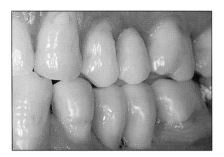

Fig 6-7 Two FRC FPDs in opposing arches. The maxillary intracoronal prosthesis exhibits low concentration of color (chroma), unlike the mandibular full-coverage prosthesis, which received internal modification to increase chroma.

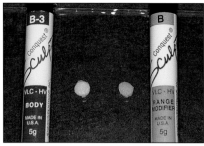

Fig 6-8 Comparison of resin with high chroma (Sculpture "B Range," Jeneric/Pentron) *(left)* and dentin shade B3.

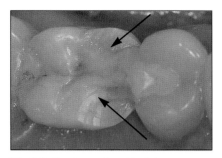

Fig 6-9 Fracture of particulate composite from the lingual cusp of the pontic on an inlay FRC FPD from the maxillary right second molar to second premolar. Sculpture/FibreKor.

Low Concentration of Color (Chroma) of Veneer, Particularly in Pontic Areas

Particulate composite "dentin" materials produced to provide the final shape of FRC prostheses may not exhibit adequate chroma. The result is a prosthesis that appears to be too "light" in appearance. It is important for the dentist and laboratory technician to be aware of this potential problem and to compare the final prosthesis shade with the actual tabs of the shade guide. If the chroma for a prosthesis is too low, the technician can begin to compensate for this problem by placing a thin layer of composite material with a high concentration of color directly over the framework or over the thin opaque layer. Examples of these concentrated materials are Sculpture (Jeneric/Pentron) "B Range" or Targis (Ivoclar) "Impulse." (Use of these materials is described in chapter 3.) Figure 6-7 shows two FRC prostheses in opposing arches. The chroma exhibited in the maxillary intracoronal FPD pontic is too low when compared to the adjacent abutment teeth, whereas the chroma in the mandibular full-coverage FPD compares more favorably to that of the adjacent natural teeth. Sculpture "B Range" was added to the framework of the mandibular FPD; this material and its similarity to dentin shade B3 are shown in Fig 6-8.

Transient Sensitivity after Cementation

When using an adhesive approach to cementation of FRC prostheses, sensitivity in the dentinal fluid flow may result from incomplete hybridization and tubule sealing in the dentin adhesive–resin cement complex.[1,2,7] Such patient postcementation sensitivity is commonly associated with drinking cold liquids and touch. Complete crown preparations present the greatest challenge in adhesive dentistry because of the number of tubules exposed; their varying orientations, combined with the remaining dentin thickness (RDT) within the preparation, make the exposed dentin tubules more difficult to seal and in general less predictable.[8,10] Proper isolation of the abutment teeth and careful application of the dentin-bonding system following manufacturer's instructions are critical to minimizing postoperative sensitivity. If, after cementation, postoperative sensitivity is present, applying a dentin primer-adhesive to the exposed margins of the retainers often can help alleviate or reduce the sensitivity. In our clinical experience, use of the multiple bottle (three-step) dentin-bonding systems seems to provide sensitivity-free adhesive cementations more consistently than do single bottle (two-step) systems, possibly as a result of better hybridization.[13]

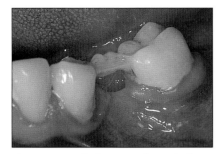

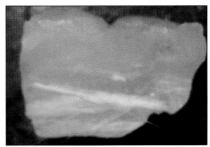

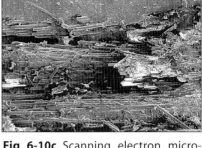

Fig 6-10a Bulk fracture of pontic from an inlay FRC FPD. Sculpture/FibreKor. This is a cohesive fracture within both the overlaying particulate composite and the FRC substructure of the pontic. Some occlusal and lingual composite remains attached to the FRC pontic substructure. This fracture was the result of too little support from the FRC framework for the pontic particulate composite. Attempts to repair this fracture will result in only short-term success since the framework design is flawed.

Fig 6-10b Detached pontic segment showing exposed glass fibers from the FRC pontic framework. (Original magnification × 20.)

Fig 6-10c Scanning electron micrograph of detached pontic with the exposed glass fibers shown in Fig 6-10b. (Original magnification × 200.) Once the glass fibers are exposed to the oral environment, they start to break down, diminishing the chances for successful long-term repair.

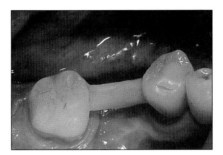

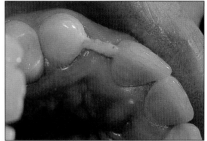

Fig 6-10d Total fracture of the veneering particulate composite from the pontic FRC framework. Targis/Vectris. (Photo courtesy of Bruce Marcucci, DDS.)

Fig 6-10e Total fracture of the veneering particulate composite from the pontic FRC framework. Sculpture/FibreKor.

Fracture of the Particulate Composite Veneer

Ease of repair of the particulate composite veneer on FRC prostheses has been suggested by manufacturers as an advantage of this technique. However, in our experience, the fracture of a section of the veneering particulate composite on an otherwise functional FRC FPD or crown can present a serious problem depending on the nature of the fracture and the design of the underlying FRC framework. During repair, aging heat- and light-cured composites exhibit a high conversion rate from intense light, pressure, and heat polymerization, limiting the number of available unbonded methacrylate groups. This reduces the likelihood of covalent bonding between the existing composite substrate and the repair resin.[5] Interfacial repair bond strengths have been shown to range anywhere from 25% to 80% of their respective substrate cohesive strengths.[4,9,11,12]

Fractures can be totally cohesive, located within the veneering particulate composite (Figs 6-9 and 6-10), or they can be both cohesive and adhesive, with the fracture extending to the FRC framework and exposing glass filler particles. The clinician must determine if the source of the problem is related to the lack of particulate composite support provided by the FRC substructure design (see framework design in chapter 3). If this appears to be the situation, our experiences have shown that a successful long-term repair probably cannot be achieved and a remake of the FPD is the only solution.

Procedures for Intraoral Repair of a Fractured Particulate Composite Veneer

Figures 6-11 to 6-13 illustrate the procedure for repairing an FRC FPD. The following materials are need for this procedure:

- Rubber dam
- Polyvinyl siloxane tray adhesive
- Microetcher with 50 μm aluminum oxide
- Silane coupling agent
- One-bottle dentin adhesive
- Flowable particulate composite resin
- Anterior/posterior restorative hybrid particulate composite resin
- Pre-impregnated FRC (Splint-It)
- Visible light–curing unit
- Composite polishing system

1. The area to be repaired is isolated with a rubber dam; sandblasted with aluminum oxide; and rinsed. Sandblasting creates a micromechanical surface to aid in the retention of the particulate composite resin repair.[3,6,11,12]
2. The repair recipient site is etched with phosphoric acid.
3. The recipient surface is silanated to chemically unite the exposed glass filler particles and fibers to the repair particulate composite resin.[6,11,12]
4. An application of a dentin adhesive is placed over the silanated surface.
5. A thin layer of flowable particulate composite is placed over the recipient site.
6. An anterior/posterior restorative particulate composite is placed and shaped to contour, or FRC strips are placed onto the recipient site to provide increased support for the repair particulate composite resin; the particulate composite is veneered over this framework.
7. The repair is polished and the occlusion checked.

Fig 6-11 Step-by-step procedure for repairing an anterior FRC FPD.

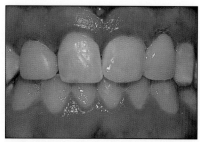

Fig 6-11a Patient at time of delivery of 3-unit direct anterior FRC FPD from the maxillary left central incisor to canine.

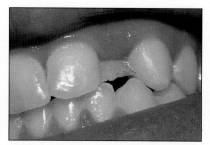

Fig 6-11b Patient presenting with fracture of labial surface of pontic, facial view. Note that the fracture is to the level of the FRC, but the framework is still intact.

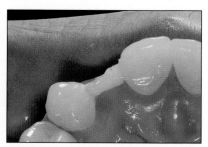

Fig 6-11c Lingual view.

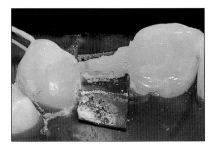

Fig 6-11d Isolation with rubber dam. The pontic ridge has been covered by a section of rubber dam that is "tacked" to the existing rubber dam by polyvinyl siloxane tray adhesive, ensuring a complete seal of the repair site.

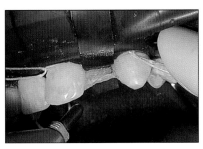

Fig 6-11e The pontic area and proximals of the adjacent retainers being abraded with 50 μm aluminum oxide. This first step in the surface preparation of the repair site aids in the retention of the particulate composite resin.

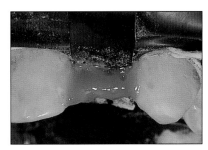

Fig 6-11f The repair site etched with 37% phosphoric acid and then rinsed.

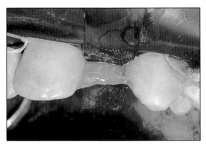

Fig 6-11g The repair site coated with silane, dentin adhesive, and a thin layer of flowable composite. It is now ready to receive the restorative hybrid composite, which will give shape to the pontic.

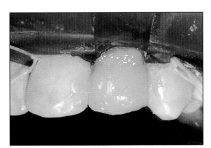

Fig 6-11h Hybrid particulate composite resin placed on the prepared recipient bed. Facial view.

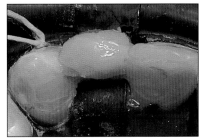

Fig 6-11i Lingual view of hybrid particulate composite resin application.

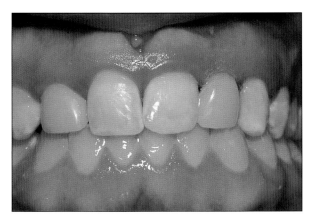

Fig 6-11j Finished pontic repair. Facial view.

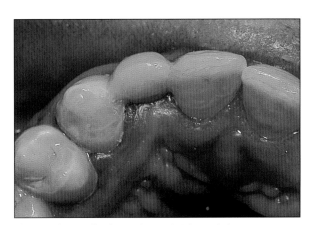

Fig 6-11k Finished pontic repair. Lingual view.

Fig 6-12 *Step-by-step procedure for repair of a posterior FRC FPD.*

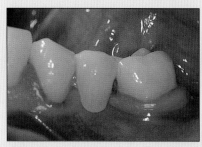
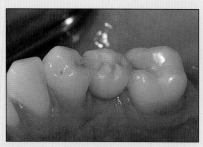

Figs 6-12a and 6-12b Facial and lingual views of posterior inlay FRC FPD at delivery.

Fig 6-12c FPD with bulk particulate composite fracture of pontic. Although the fracture was at the level of the FRC pontic framework, it did not expose any glass fibers.

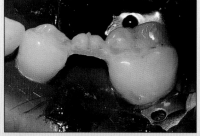
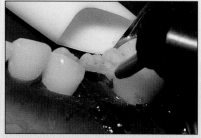
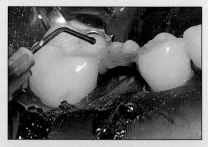

Fig 6-12d Rubber dam application with pontic ridge covered for complete isolation of the repair site.

Fig 6-12e Air abrasion to start the surface preparation of the repair site.

Fig 6-12f Etching of repair site with 37% phosphoric acid.

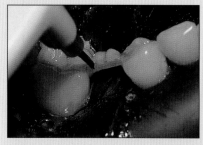
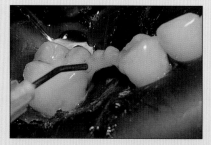
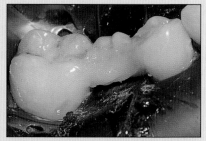

Fig 6-12g Repair site being silanated. A dentin adhesive is then applied.

Fig 6-12h Flowable composite resin being applied prior to the restorative particulate composite resin.

Fig 6-12i Initial increment of particulate composite resin initiating the recovery of the pontic shape.

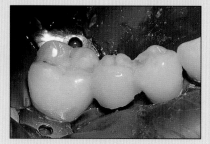
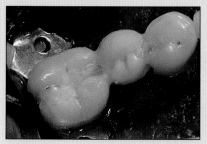

Fig 6-12j Finished pontic repair, facial view.

Fig 6-12k Finished pontic repair, occlusal view. This repair was predictably short-lived because of the lack of FRC pontic framework support in the initial design of the FPD.

Fig 6-13 *Step-by-step procedure for repair of a posterior FRC FPD using additional FRC.*

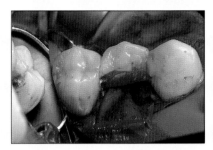

Fig 6-13a Fractured pontic on a full-coverage FRC FPD. The fracture is at the level of the FRC framework, but it does not involve exposure of the glass fibers.

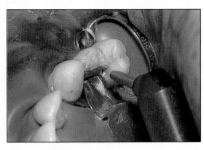

Fig 6-13b Small Class III preparations placed into the proximal areas of the retainers at the level of the FRC. These serve as a platform for placement of the ends of the FRC material, which will increase the framework support for the pontic particulate composite repair. Air abrasion is performed to initiate the surface preparation of the repair site.

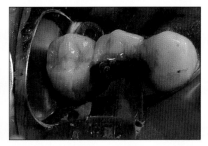

Fig 6-13c The repair site etched with phosphoric acid.

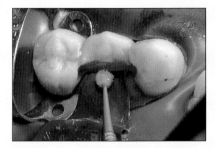

Fig 6-13d The repair site, which has undergone application of silane and a dentin adhesive.

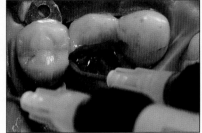

Fig 6-13e A flowable composite resin being placed onto the repair site and into the Class III preparations to aid in tacking the preresinated FRC material in place.

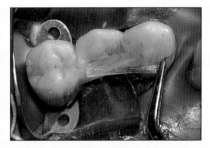

Fig 6-13f Preresinated FRC strips being added to the repair site and then light cured to provide an increase in structural support for the veneering particulate composite resin. This approach is an attempt to correct the design deficiency of the original FRC framework in the pontic area.

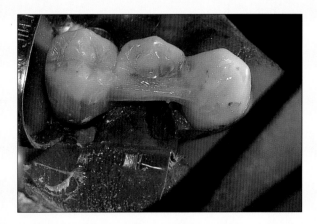

Fig 6-13g The completed extension of the FRC framework prior to addition of the hybrid restorative particulate composite resin, which will restore shape and function to the missing pontic segment.

Fig 6-14 Recementation of a loose inlay design FRC FPD.

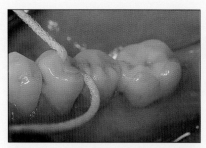

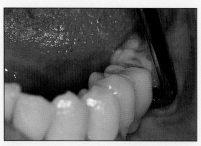

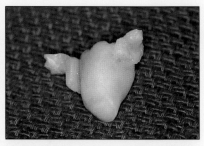

Fig 6-14a Posterior inlay FRC FPD with a loose retainer on the premolar abutment. The distal retainer is still adhesively attached to the molar abutment. This FPD can be salvaged if it can be removed intact and successfully recemented.

Fig 6-14b A crown remover used to gently initiate a fracture within the luting composite resin surrounding the molar retainer, so as to permit removal of the FPD while avoiding fracturing any section of the bonded retainer.

Fig 6-14c Inlay FPD successfully removed intact. The tissue side of the retainers are air abraded to remove any residual luting composite resin and to provide a micromechanical surface for the new luting composite resin.

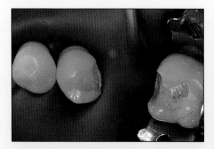

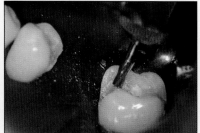

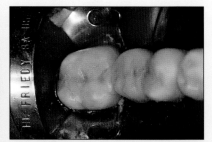

Fig 6-14d Appearance of the abutment teeth preparations. Some residual luting composite resin remains in sections of each preparation.

Fig 6-14e The residual luting composite resin being cleaned from the preparations. Care must be taken to avoid altering the shape of the preparations, since that would decrease the accuracy of fit of the FPD retainers.

Fig 6-14f Inlay FPD recemented.

Debonding of the Retainer

Problems associated with the adhesive retention of an FRC FPD may present in two forms: total loss of attachment from both abutment teeth, or loss of attachment from one of the two abutments, leaving the FPD in the mouth. If there is no damage, either to the FPD or to the abutment teeth, the FRC can be recemented by repeating the steps described in chapter 3. Recementation of a loose inlay design FRC FPD is shown in Fig 6-14.

References

1. Brannstrom M. The hydrodynamic theory of dentinal pain: Sensation in preparations, caries, and dentinal crack syndrome. J Endod 1986;12:453–457.

2. Brannstrom M. The cause of postrestorative sensitivity and its prevention J Endod 1986;12:475–481.

3. Bouschlicher MR, Reinhardt JW, Vargas MA. Surface treatment techniques for resin composite repair. Am J Dent 1997;10:279–283.

4. Ciba K, Hosoda H, Fusayama T. The addition of an adhesive composite resin to the same material: Bond strength and clinical techniques. J Prosthet Dent 1989;61:669–675.

5. Heymann HO, Haywood VB, Andreaus SB, Bayne SC. Bonding agent strengths with processed composite resin veneers. Dent Mater 1987;3:121–124.

6. Imamura GM, Reinhardt JW, Boyer DB, Swift EJ. Enhancement of resin bonding to heat-cured composite resin. Oper Dent 1996;21:249–256.

7. Pashley DH. Dentin permeability, dentin sensitivity, and treatment through tubule occlusion. J Endod 1986; 12:465–474.

8. Pashley EL, Comer RW, Simpson MD, Horner JA, Pashley DH, Caughman WF. Dentin permeability: Sealing the dentin in crown preparations. Oper Dent 1992; 17:13–20.

9. Puckett AD, Holder R, O'Hara JW. Strength of posterior composite repairs using different composite/bonding agent combinations. Oper Dent 1991;16:136–140.

10. Richardson D, Tao L, Pashley DH. Dentin permeability: Effects of crown preparation. Int J Prosthodont 1991;4:219–225.

11. Rosentritt M, Behr M, Leibrock A, Handel G, Friedl K-H. Intraoral repair of fiber-reinforced composite fixed partial dentures. J Prosthet Dent 1998;79:393–398.

12. Turner CW, Meiers JC. Repair of an aged, contaminated indirect composite resin with a direct, visible-light-cured composite resin. Oper Dent 1993;18:187–194.

13. Van Meerbeek B, Yoshida Y, Snauwaert J, Hellemans L, Lambrechts P, Vanherle G, Wakasa K, Pashley DH. Hybridization effectiveness of a two-step versus a three-step smear layer removing adhesive system examined correlatiely by TEM and AFM. J Adhes Dent 1999;1:7–23.

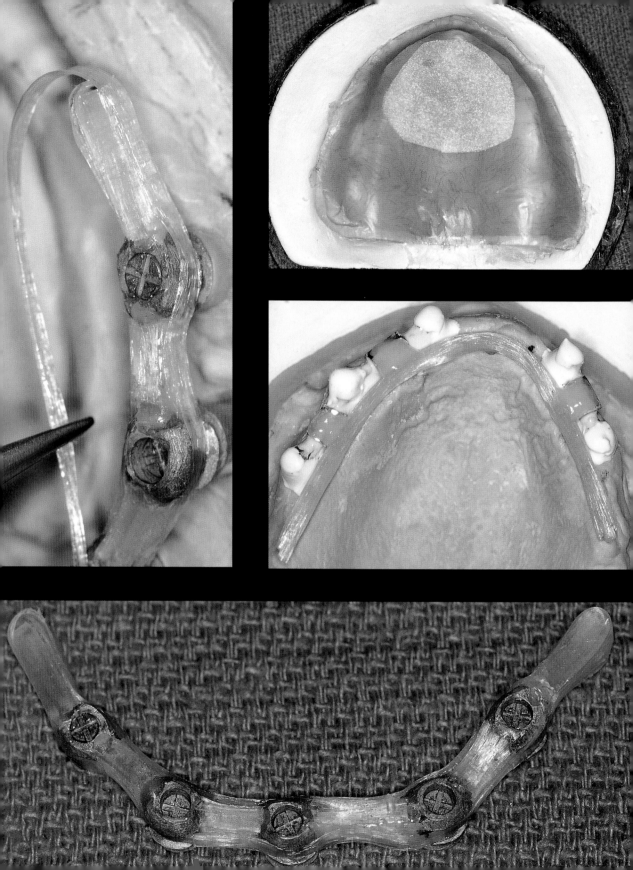

Future Applications of FRC

■ Previous chapters have shown that fiber-reinforced composites (FRCs) can be used to fabricate tooth-supported fixed prostheses. Both chairside and laboratory techniques have been used with success to create these restorations. Fiber-reinforced composites are also used to make posts and space maintainers and to repair acrylic resin prostheses and appliances. These represent only the first of many applications of this material in dentistry. Presented below are some concepts and techniques that may become popular in dentistry in the near future.

Implants

Dental implants have become a standard of care for tooth replacement in both partially and completely edentulous arches. Implants are routinely restored with overdentures, fixed partial dentures (FPDs), or hybrid (fixed-removable) prostheses. Short edentulous spans can be successfully restored with fiber-reinforced FPDs (Fig 7-1). Despite the short-term success that has been achieved in restoring short edentulous spans, the standard metallic or cylinder form abutment is less than ideal because of its esthetic and bonding limitations and because it has proven unacceptable for restoring a hybrid type of prosthesis.[1]

Fig 7-1 *Three-unit FRC FPD restoring ITI implants with cementable-type abutments.*

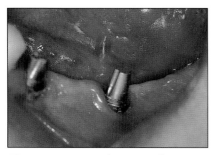 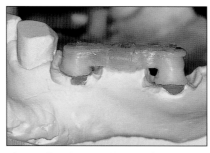 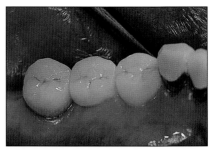

Fig 7-1a Intraoral view of ITI ce-mentable-type abutments.

Fig 7-1b Fiber-reinforced framework for 3-unit FPD on implants.

Fig 7-1c Intraoral view of cemented FRC FPD.

The standard technique for restoring a multiple-unit implant-supported prosthesis is to use a cast metal framework. A prosthesis made with an FRC framework and corresponding abutments and cylinders has several advantages over the standard techniques:

1. The laboratory procedure for creating a fiber-reinforced framework takes less time than current methods.
2. The fewer labor hours combined with lower material costs results in a prosthesis that is less expensive than its traditional counterpart.
3. The need for sectioning and soldering, as with long-span metal frameworks, is eliminated.
4. The overlaying suprastructure (whether polymethyl methacrylate [PMMA] for a hybrid prosthesis or composite veneers for an FPD) will mechanically and chemically bond to the FRC framework. Polymethyl methacrylate and porcelain do not chemically bond to the metal framework currently used for these prostheses.
5. The use of composite resin materials has distinct advantages over porcelain veneers: they are less brittle, they cause no wear to the opposing dentition, they may be repaired, and so forth.
6. It is not necessary to block out the metal framework with opaque materials, so the final result has an even greater esthetic potential.

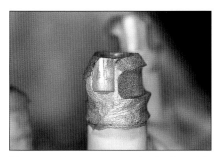

Fig 7-2a Prototype metal cylinder with proximal and buccal grooves to retain, support, and aid in positioning of the FRC framework.

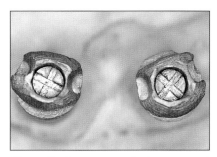

Fig 7-2b Prototype cylinder screwed into place on an ITI octabutment.

Prototype metal cylinders have been developed by the authors for use in multiple-unit prostheses supported by several implants (Fig 7-2). These cylinders, which are screwed into the standard abutment, are designed to support, position, and retain the FRC framework. Additional cylinder and abutment designs have been conceptualized, including an all-ceramic cylinder, a polymer-coated cylinder, and a UCLA-type abutment. All of these designs have the potential to enhance the structural integrity and esthetic possibilities of the final restoration.

In conjunction with the prototype metal cylinders, the authors have also developed a method for fabricating a successful hybrid prosthesis supported by multiple implants in the edentulous arch (Fig 7-3).

Further laboratory and clinical development are needed before these materials and techniques will be readily available to the practitioner, but this area shows great promise.

Fig 7-3 *Laboratory procedures for the fabrication of a hybrid-type prosthesis.*

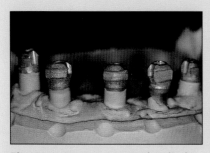

Fig 7-3a Prototype metal cylinders are screwed into lab analogue abutments on the master cast.

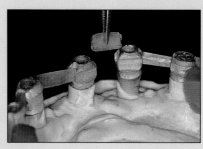

Fig 7-3b Prefabricated bars of FRC are placed so as to connect the cylinders.

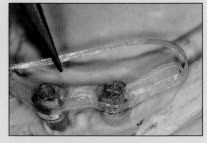

Fig 7-3c After the bars of FRC have been polymerized, continuous strips of FRC are wrapped into the buccal grooves around the entire framework longitudinally and bonded to the bars of FRC.

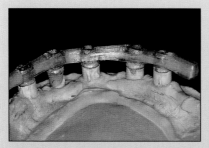

Fig 7-3d The final framework is polymerized. (Note: future models will incorporate a supporting ledge on the distalmost abutments to support the cantilever.)

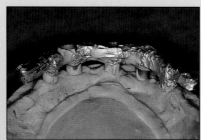

Fig 7-3e After final polymerization, all FRC surfaces and cylinders are covered with aluminum foil.

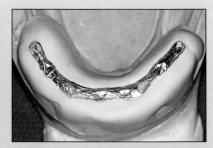

Fig 7-3f A polyvinyl siloxane putty is then used to create a matrix surrounding all nonocclusal surfaces of the framework.

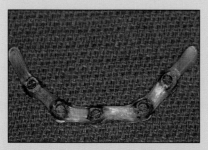

Fig 7-3g The FRC framework is removed.

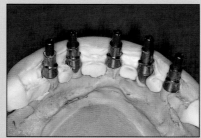

Fig 7-3h Aluminum provisional cylinders are screwed onto the master cast to make the verfication stent, which is then brought to the patient's mouth to ensure accuracy of the master cast.

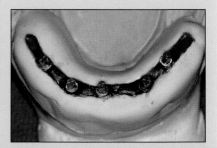

Fig 7-3i The verification stent is made by pouring pattern resin into the putty matrix.

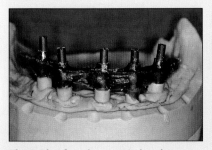

Fig 7-3j After the matrix has been removed, the verification stent will be removed from the cast and tried in the patient's mouth.

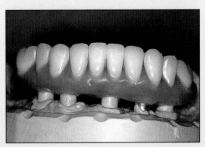

Fig 7-3k After the accuracy of the master cast has been confirmed, the verification stent is used as the foundation for setting the denture teeth.

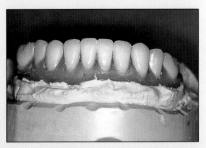

Fig 7-3l The finalized denture waxup is brought to the apical edge of the aluminum cylinder. Everything below this finish line is blocked out with polyvinyl siloxane putty or plaster.

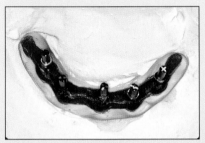

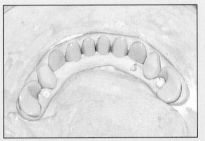

Figs 7-3m and 7-3n The denture setup is then flasked and boiled out, leaving the verification stent on one side of the flask and the denture teeth on the other.

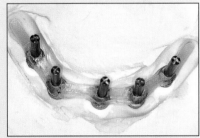

Fig 7-3o The verfication stent is removed, and the FRC framework is replaced on the flasked master cast.

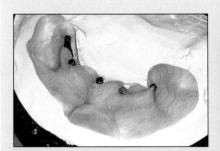

Fig 7-3p Acrylic resin is then packed and the prosthesis is polymerized, finished, and polished following standard denture-processing techniques.

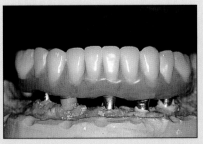

Figs 7-3q and 7-3r The final restoration, shown on and off the master cast.

Fig 7-4 Sample fiber-reinforced framework in an implant-supported bar overdenture.

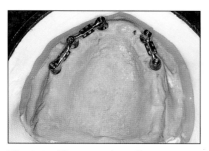
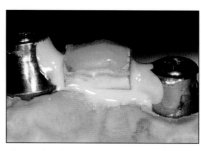
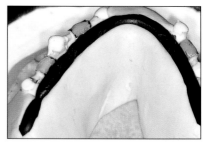

Fig 7-4a The retentive clips are connected to the bar, and a flowable composite is syringed into the mechanical retention on top of the clip that retains it in the denture and connects it to the FRC framework.

Fig 7-4b The retentive portion of the clips are blocked out to ensure that they remain patent during final processing of the resin.

Fig 7-4c A rope of inlay wax is waxed to the master cast to create a pattern for the FRC framework. A silicone putty is adapted around the matrix to form a trough to stabilize the FRC during polymerization.

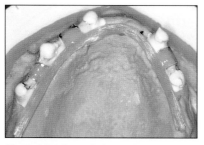
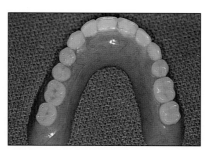

Fig 7-4d A bar of FRC in the appropriate length and width is then secured to the retentive clips by flowable composite. The entire framework is then polymerized.

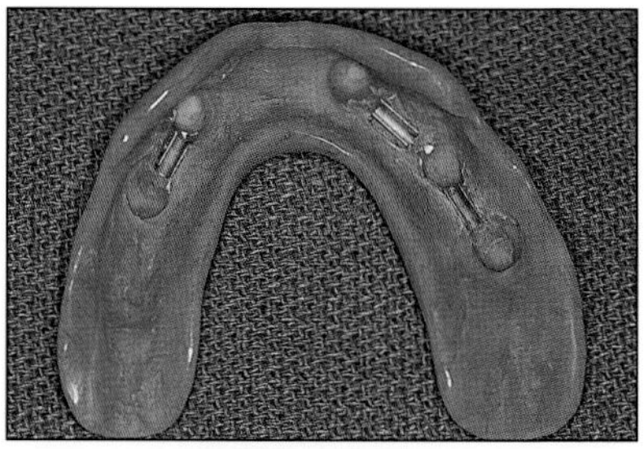

Figs 7-4e and 7-4f The denture is processed, cured, and finished using standard techniques, resulting in a virtually metal-free reinforced prosthesis.

Overdenture Frameworks

Overdentures retained by implants or with attachments to natural dentition are routinely reinforced with a metal framework. This metal framework is time-consuming to fabricate, costly, unesthetic, and requires the use of alloys that can present health dangers to the technicians who routinely use them.[13,14] The authors have developed a method for creating an FRC framework to replace the traditional metal framework for overdentures (Fig 7-4). This process requires no special abutments or cylinders other than those routinely used to restore an overdenture with a metal framework.

Denture Reinforcement

Fractures of maxillary complete dentures opposing a natural dentition are very common, and they are being seen with increasing frequency when opposing an implant-supported prosthesis (Fig 7-5). A broken denture is a predicament dreaded by patients and clinicians alike. Dentures fracture as a result of both impact and flexural fatigue.[8,10,18,21] When a patient has a history of fractured dentures or presents with opposing natural teeth or implants in the mandible, a reinforced denture should be considered.

Over the years, attempts have been made to reinforce denture resins (polymethyl methacry-

Fig 7-5 *Maxillary dentures most commonly fracture through the frenal notch and are associated with an intact opposing dentition.*

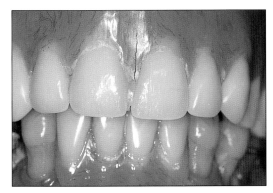

Fig 7-5a Fractured denture opposing a removable partial denture.

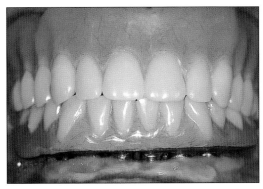

Fig 7-5b Fractured denture opposing an implant-supported prosthesis.

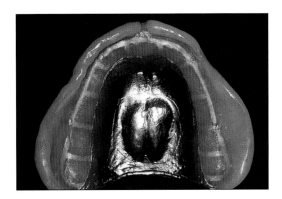

Fig 7-6 A maxillary denture with a metal-reinforced palate used in cases of repeated fractures.

late with metal wires and plates,[4,9,16,20] carbon fibers,[5,12,17] aramid fibers,[2,15] polyethylene fibers,[3,11] and glass fibers.[6,7,19] While it has been demonstrated that PMMA can be significantly reinforced, a predictable, convenient, and esthetic technique for reinforcement of PMMA has not been found.

In fact, the method accepted by many dentists when repeated fractures occur is to fabricate the denture with a metal framework (Fig 7-6). Though reliable, this technique is also expensive, unesthetic, and time-consuming, and does not allow the denture to be relined or rebased if necessary.

As noted in earlier chapters, the superior flexure strength of a glass FRC, combined with the ability of its resinous matrix to both uniformly wet the fibers and chemically bond to

the parent resin, makes it an ideal material for resin reinforcement. Furthermore, glass FRCs have been shown to have significantly greater flexural properties than unreinforced PMMA.[22]

Initially, only strips of light-polymerized FRC were used for denture reinforcement. While this material is effective for chairside repairs, it is not ideal for incorporating during processing. When reinforcing a complete denture, the use of light polymerization and the handling and cutting of the individual FRC strips are cumbersome additions to the processing technique. At the packing stage, the individual strips must be placed and then polymerized with visible light before the flasks can be closed (Fig 7-7). These extra procedures encroach upon the working time of the denture resin and require a light-curing unit.

Fig 7-7 *Dentures reinforced with light-polymerized strips of FRC require multiple additional steps during processing, including cutting, tacking down, and light curing.*

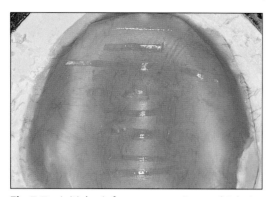

Fig 7-7a Initial reinforcements using multiple individual strips of FRC.

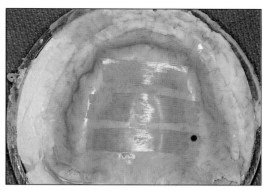

Fig 7-7b Later reinforcements using wider strips of FRC.

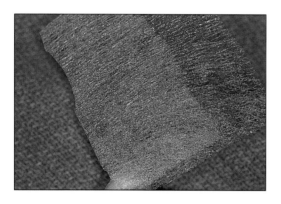

Fig 7-8 A sheet of heat-polymerized FRC, which eliminates many of the earlier difficulties associated with light-polymerized strips of FRC for reinforcement.

It is clear that any reinforcing material must be easily incorporated into standard denture-processing techniques to be adopted for routine and successful use. As a solution to these problems, a heat-polymerized, woven sheet of FRC has been developed that can be easily incorporated into standard denture-processing practice (Fig 7-8). Although the technique for using this material is shown, this material is not commercially available at this time.

The technique developed for the fabrication of a fiber-reinforced denture with a woven sheet of heat-polymerized FRC requires no additional procedures prior to the processing stage. At the packing stage, a precut sheet of FRC is incorporated between the halves of the denture resin just before the flask is closed and placed into the curing tank (Fig 7-9). Once the denture is removed from the curing tank, it is polished and delivered using standard techniques.

Summary

The use of FRCs in both implant dentistry and removable prosthodontics has broad potential. The strength, esthetics, and versatility of these materials will allow for the development of new applications as well as the enhancement of existing techniques. The future holds great promise for fiber-reinforced composites in all areas of clinical and laboratory dentistry.

Fig 7-9 *Fabrication of a heat-polymerized fiber-reinforced denture.*

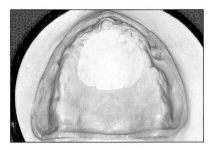

Fig 7-9a After a denture is flasked and boiled out, a template for the dimensions of the woven FRC is made using any convenient material. In this case, a paper towel was cut to cover the appropriate area.

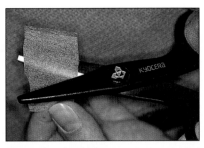

Fig 7-9b Using ceramic scissors and the template, the sheet of woven FRC is cut to the appropriate size.

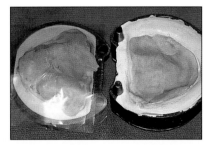

Fig 7-9c Unlike conventional trial packing, equal amounts of denture resin are placed against the master cast and against the denture teeth with acetate sheets dividing the two halves.

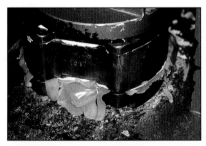

Fig 7-9d The flask is then closed under pressure and the excess resin is removed.

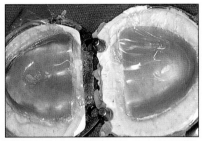

Fig 7-9e When the flask is opened, resin should cover both "halves" of the denture to completely embed the FRC sheet within the denture resin. If stone is evident on one side, resin must be removed from one half of the flask and added to the other half and trial packed again.

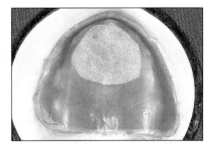

Fig 7-9f Once the resin is equally divided, the sheet of woven FRC is placed.

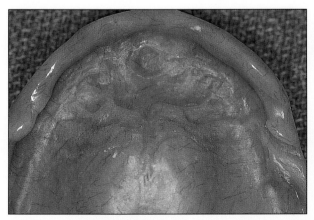
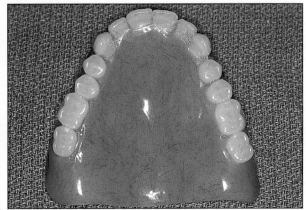

Figs 7-9g and 7-9h After standard polymerization in the curing tank, the denture is finished and polished using conventional techniques.

References

1. Bergendal T, Ekstrand K, Karlsson U. Evaluation of implant-supported carbon/graphite fiber-reinforced poly (methyl methacrylate) prostheses. A longitudinal multicenter study. Clin Oral Implants Res 1995;6:246–253.

2. Berrong JM, Weed RW, Young JM. Fracture resistance of kevlar-reinforced poly(methacrylate) resin: A preliminary study. Int J Prosthodont 1990;3:391–395.

3. Braden M, Davy KWM, Parker S, Ladizesky NH, Ward IM. Denture base poly(methacrylate) reinforced with ultrahigh modulus polyethylene fibers. Br Dent J 1988; 164:109–113.

4. Carroll C, von Fraunhofer J. Wire reinforcement of acrylic resin prostheses. J Prosthet Dent 1984;52:639–641.

5. Ekstrand K, Ruyter I, Wellendorf H. Carbon/graphite fiber reinforced poly(methylmethacrylate): Properties under dry and wet conditions. J Biomed Mater Res 1987; 21:1065–1080.

6. Freilich MA, Karmaker AC, Burstone CJ, Goldberg AJ. Flexure strength of fiber-reinforced composites designed for prosthodontic application [abstract 999]. J Dent Res 1997;76:138.

7. Goldberg AJ, Freilich MA, Haser KA, Audi JH. Flexure properties and fiber architecture of commercial fiber reinforced composites [abstract 967]. J Dent Res 1998;77:226.

8. Johnston EP, Nicholls JI, Smith DE. Flexure fatigue of 10 commonly used denture base resins. J Prosthet Dent 1981;46:478–483.

9. Kawano F, Miyamoto M, Tada N, Matsumoto N. Reinforcement of acrylic resin denture base with NI-Cr alloy plate. Int J Prosthodont 1990;3:484–488.

10. Kelly E. Fatigue failure in denture base polymers. J Prosthet Dent 1969;21:257–266.

11. Ladizesky NH, Ho CF, Chow TW. Reinforcement of complete denture bases with continuous high performance polyethylene fibers. J Prosthet Dent 1992; 68:934–939.

12. Manley TR, Bowman AJ, Cook M. Denture bases reinforced with carbon fibers. Br Dent J 1979;146:25.

13. Moffa JP. Allergic response to nickel containing dental alloys [abstract 107]. J Dent Res 1977;56:1378.

14. Morris HF. Veterans Administration Cooperative Studies Project No. 147. IV. Biocompatibility of base metal alloys. J Dent 1987;58:1.

15. Mullarky R. Aramid fiber reinforcement of acrylic appliances. J Clin Orthod 1985;19:655–658.

16. Ruffino A. Effect of steel strengtheners on fracture resistance of the acrylic resin complete denture base. J Prosthet Dent 1985;54:75–78.

17. Schreiber C. Polymethylmethacrylate reinforced with carbon fibers. Br Dent J 1971;130:29–30.

18. Smith DC. The acrylic denture: Mechanical evaluation of mid-line fracture. Br Dent J 1961;110:257–267.

19. Solnit G. The effect of methyl methacrylate reinforcement with silane-treated and untreated glass fibers. J Prosthet Dent 1991;66:310–314.

20. Vallittu P. Reinforcement of acrylic resin denture base material with metal or fiber strengtheners. J Oral Rehabil 1992;19:225–230.

21. Vallittu PK, Lassila VP, Lappalainen R. Number and type of damages of removable dentures in two cities in Finland. Acta Odontol Scand 1993;51:363–369.

22. Vallittu PK. Flexural properties of acrylic resin polymers reinforced with unidirectional and woven glass fibers. J Prosthet Dent 1999;81:318–326.

Index